10-31-06

MW01482372

PR YOURSELF FROM THE FLU AND OTHER INFECTIONS

Contributing Writers:
Laurie L. Dove
Michele Price Mann

Consultant:
Larry Lutwick, M.D.

Publications International, Ltd.

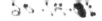

Contributing Writers:

Laurie L. Dove is an award-winning Kansas-based journalist and author whose work has been published internationally. Dove is a dedicated consumer advocate who specializes in writing about health, parenting, fitness, and travel. An active member of the National Federation of Press Women, Dove also is the former owner of a parenting magazine and a weekly newspaper. Learn more about Dove and her current projects by visiting www.lauriedove.com.

Michele Price Mann is a freelance writer who has written for such publications as *Weight Watchers Magazine* and *Southern Living* magazine and was assistant health and fitness editor at *Cooking Light* magazine. Learning and writing about health issues has been a professional passion for Mann.

Consultant:

Larry Lutwick, M.D., is a professor of medicine at the State University of New York-Downstate Medical School in Brooklyn, New York, and director of infectious diseases, Veterans Affairs New York Harbor Health Care System, Brooklyn Campus. He is also bacterial diseases moderator for the real-time online infectious diseases surveillance system, Program for Monitoring Emerging Diseases (ProMED-mail). Lutwick has written more than 100 medical articles and 15 book chapters and has edited two books about infectious diseases.

Illustrations: Jeff Moores

Unless otherwise noted, all scripture quotations are taken from the New Revised Standard Version of the Bible, copyright © 1989, by the Division of Christian Education of the National Council of the Churches of Christ in the United States of America. Used by permission. All rights reserved.

This book is for informational purposes and is not intended to provide medical advice. Neither Publications International, Ltd., nor the authors, consultant, or publisher take responsibility for any possible consequences from any treatment, procedure, exercise, dietary modification, action, or application of medication or preparation by any person reading or following the information in this book. The publication of this book does not constitute the practice of medicine, and this book does not attempt to replace your physician or other health-care provider. Before undertaking any course of treatment, the authors, consultant, editors, and publisher advise the reader to check with a physician or other health-care provider.

The brand-name products mentioned in this publication are trademarks or service marks of their respective companies. The mention of any product in this publication does not constitute an endorsement by the respective proprietors of Publications International, Ltd., nor does it constitute an endorsement by any of these companies that their products should be used in the manner represented in this publication.

Louis Weber, CEO
Publications International, Ltd.
7373 North Cicero Avenue
Lincolnwood, Illinois 60712

Permission is never granted for commercial purposes.

ISBN-13: 978-1-4127-1380-1
ISBN-10: 1-4127-1380-3

Manufactured in U.S.A.

8 7 6 5 4 3 2 1

Contents

Introduction

Commonsense Defense Against Tiny Terrors

Your body's immune system battles disease-causing bacteria, viruses, and parasites every day. You're not aware of this ongoing warfare because most of the time the immune system quietly vanquishes these threats to keep you healthy. However, even a strong immune system can't defend you if you don't take some basic but essential measures to protect yourself against these tiny armies of illness.

Protect Yourself from the Flu and Other Infections examines more than 70 diseases caused by these invisible invaders that target every part of your body. The profile of each one explains the culprit behind the infection, how you contract it, its symptoms, its most likely victims, and, most important, the practical defensive measures you can take to protect yourself and your family.

This book discusses smart and simple strategies to avoid a variety of infectious diseases, but keep in mind that the information provided here is intended to complement, not replace, proper medical care and the advice of a health-care professional. Only he or she knows your exact medical history and any additional risks you might face. So if you have any questions, be sure to bring them up at your next appointment. In the meantime, though, use this handy guide to fortify your defenses against the tiny squadrons of sickness that surround us all.

Chapter 1 In the News

For years, the saying in television newsrooms was "If it bleeds, it leads." These days, it might be "If it scares, it airs." Infectious diseases, such as bird flu and mad cow disease, are getting loads of press, but what are your real risks? Read on for practical tips to protect yourself from infection.

AIDS (Acquired Immune Deficiency Syndrome)

CULPRIT Human immunodeficiency virus (HIV) causes AIDS, which is the term used to describe the later, potentially more serious, stages of HIV infection.

INFECTION INFO HIV damages the immune system and destroys the body's CD4 T lymphocytes (T cells), one of many types of white blood cells the body uses to fight disease. T cells help the immune system "identify" foreign organisms that should be attacked. Thus, when the T cells are destroyed, it's like being defended by a leaderless army that is easily defeated.

A person can be infected with HIV for ten years or even longer without showing any symptoms. However, in most cases, during that time the virus is attacking the immune system and destroying T cells. By the time HIV damages enough cells to bring on full-blown AIDS, many of the typical symptoms can be present: weight loss, sporadic fevers, fatigue, swollen lymph nodes, diarrhea, and opportunistic infections such as certain types of pneumonia. Rare cancers and infections of the kidneys, digestive system, and brain can also develop.

HIV is passed from person to person by direct contact with blood or other body fluids through activities like unprotected vaginal, anal, or oral sexual contact with an infected person or through sharing syringes or needles during intravenous drug use or tattooing. HIV-infected mothers can transmit the virus to their children during pregnancy, during childbirth, or through breast milk. Before 1985, HIV was passed through blood transfusions. Today, however, according to the American Red Cross, donated blood is routinely screened for HIV, making the risk of acquiring HIV through a blood transfusion less than one in 1.5 million.

A great deal of progress has been made in the nearly 30 years since HIV and AIDS were first recognized. Although HIV infection is a terminal illness with no cure or vaccine, people today can live with HIV for years, and they might not develop AIDS, thanks to a combination of medications. With treatment, HIV/AIDS can be considered a chronic disease like high blood pressure or diabetes in many people.

However, HIV infection is a major threat in the developing world, where treatment is often unavailable. According to the Joint United Nations Programme on HIV/AIDS, 24.5 million of the 38.6 million people in the world who are infected with HIV live in sub-Saharan Africa.

WHO'S AT RISK People who share needles for intravenous drug use, tattooing, or body piercing have a higher risk of contracting HIV, as do those who have unprotected sex. As mentioned earlier, children born to HIV-infected mothers are also at risk of contracting the virus.

DEFENSIVE MEASURES HIV cannot be spread through casual contact. This means you can't contract HIV from someone who is infected with the disease by touching common surfaces, hugging, crying, or even kissing with a closed mouth (according to the available scientific evidence, the risk of transmitting HIV even through open-mouth kissing is very low). There are also ways you can protect yourself from this virus:

■ According to the Centers for Disease Control and Prevention (CDC), one of the best ways to avoid HIV and AIDS is to abstain from sexual intercourse or to keep sexual activity within the confines of a long-term, monogamous relationship where both partners have been tested for HIV (and it's a good idea to be tested for other sexually transmitted diseases, too).

■ If you do have sex, use a condom.

■ Don't share hygiene items that may come into contact with blood, such as a toothbrush or razor.

■ If you are getting a tattoo or a body piercing, don't share needles. Be sure you are working with a reputable tattoo artist or piercer who follows strict sanitary guidelines.

■ Anyone who uses intravenous drugs or receives any kind of injection should use a clean syringe each time. Never share syringes because infections, including HIV, can be passed among people through them.

■ If you are pregnant or would like to become pregnant, talk with your physician about getting an HIV test. If you test positive, there are medications that can reduce the chance of passing HIV to your baby.

■ If you're HIV-positive, tell your sexual partners about your infection so they can be tested.

BIOTERRORISM 101

Bioterrorism has received a great deal of attention recently due to terrorist attacks in the United States and other parts of the world. Could infections be used effectively as weapons, and if so, what should we be worried about?

The infections that pose the highest risk if weaponized are called category A agents. According to the Centers for Disease Control and Prevention (CDC), category A agents have the highest risk because they can be easily spread, can result in high death rates and have a major impact on public health, can cause social panic, and require special action for public health preparedness. The CDC classifies other, lower-risk infections as category B and category C risks.

The category A agents are anthrax, botulism, plague, small-pox, tularemia, and viral hemorrhagic fevers (such as Ebola virus). All these infections occur naturally, usually sporadically, in certain areas or circumstances throughout the world. Their use in biowarfare could cause them to occur in an epidemic, in forms less commonly found in nature, and/or in areas where the disease does not normally occur. (Three other boxes in this chapter contain information about these specific agents.)

Antibiotic-Associated Colitis (Pseudomembranous Colitis, C. diff Colitis)

CULPRIT The bacterium *Clostridium difficile* is to blame for antibiotic-associated colitis.

INFECTION INFO Antibiotic-associated colitis is caused by toxins in the intestines after a person undergoes antibiotic treatment. After antibiotics kill off some of the other competing bacteria, the usually harmless spores of *C. difficile* germinate, growing rapidly and releasing toxins that damage the intestinal wall.

Although all antibiotics have the potential to create this situation, the most common culprits are clindamycin, ampicillin, amoxicillin, and all antibiotics in the cephalosporin family. Certain cancer chemotherapy drugs can also cause the disease.

The disease's most prominent symptom, diarrhea, usually begins five to ten days (or longer) after starting antibiotic treatment. Other indications include abdominal cramps, fever, fatigue, and an elevated white blood cell count. Once the antibiotic that caused the symptoms is no longer in the body, mild cases of antibiotic-associated colitis can pass without complication (and without specific treatment) in about two weeks, as long as dehydration is prevented. Sometimes, people are given a different antibiotic to control the growth of *C. difficile* or even supplements that contain microorganisms to help replace some of the intestine's "good" bacteria.

In 2004, an outbreak of more severe *C. difficile* disease began primarily in Canada and England. This strain of the organism is a mutant that produces ten to 20 times more toxin than other strains and has even occurred in people who have not received antibiotics or cancer chemotherapy.

About 50 percent of people with antibiotic-associated colitis will develop a severe complication called pseudomembranous enterocolitis, in which white blood cells, mucus, and the protein that causes blood to clot (fibrin) are excreted in the stool. If this

BIOTERRORISM AGENTS: ANTHRAX AND BOTULISM

Anthrax:

- Caused by infection with and toxins produced by the bacterium *Bacillus anthracis*
- Transmitted through spores in the environment
- Natural infection is usually a skin infection with an ulcer
- Natural cases are very rare in the United States; most occur in Asia and Africa
- Weaponized versions of anthrax could be spread through inhalation
- Does not spread from person to person
- Can be treated with antibiotics and vaccine
- Without treatment, inhaled anthrax has a mortality rate close to 100 percent; if properly treated, the mortality rate is about 50 percent

Botulism:

- Caused by nerve toxins that are created by the bacterium *Clostridium botulinum*
- Usually associated with improper home canning or other food-preservation methods
- Causes paralysis that can affect breathing and may necessitate respiratory support
- When weaponized, the toxin may be spread in foods, water, or inhaled forms
- Many cases at once would signify use as a bioweapon
- Can be treated with antitoxin; a vaccine is being developed
- Without treatment, botulism has a mortality of 100 percent if respiratory failure occurs; when treated with antitoxin and respiratory support, mortality rate is about 6 percent in the United States

happens, a high fever, nausea, dehydration, low blood pressure, and even a tear in the wall of the large intestine could occur.

WHO'S AT RISK Those 60 and older have an increased risk of developing antibiotic-associated colitis because they are more likely to have *C. difficile* spores already present in their intestines. People who are severely ill or who have weakened immune systems, as well as hospitalized people, are also more susceptible.

DEFENSIVE MEASURES The best way to protect yourself from antibiotic-associated colitis is to stay healthy and avoid bacterial infections so you don't have to take antibiotics. This means washing your hands, eating a balanced and nutritious diet, exercising, and taking a daily multivitamin. If you do contract antibiotic-associated colitis, being in good health can help reduce your chance of developing complications and can mean a shorter bout with the illness. *C. difficile* spores can survive in excreted stools and be spread to others, so hand washing and proper disposal of diapers is especially important.

Because this disease is common in hospitals, health-care organizations are trying to control the inappropriate use of antibiotics.

Bird Flu
(Avian Influenza, Avian Influenza A H5N1)

CULPRIT Avian influenza is an infection caused by certain new strains of influenza virus that live in the intestines of birds.

INFECTION INFO Birds spread avian influenza viruses in feces, mucus, and body fluids. In birds, symptoms can be mild, but at its most severe (especially in poultry), avian influenza attacks multiple internal organs and causes death in about two days.

There are many different subtypes of bird flu viruses, and most don't affect people. However, some subtypes, most commonly the strain known as avian influenza A H5N1, can infect humans. When a person contracts bird flu, symptoms mimic human influenza complaints, including cough, muscle aches, fever, and sore throat, but the infection might worsen and cause pneumonia, breathing difficulties, and even death. In documented cases of human infection with H5N1, half of those infected have died.

Although avian influenza viruses can spread from bird to bird and bird to person, they rarely spread from person to person, according to the National Institutes of Health. Importantly, as of this printing, the virus has not caused chains of infection from person to person, and no cases of H5N1 bird flu have been reported in the United States. So why all the fear? The U.S. Department of State predicts the avian influenza virus could soon arrive in the Western Hemisphere, thanks to bird migration and the possibility of transportation of infected poultry.

But the bigger danger comes from the nature of viruses. The influenza virus is very dynamic and has the ability to change quickly, especially when different strains mix with each other. Experts are concerned that a bird flu virus could mutate into a highly contagious form that could be passed person to person.

People haven't developed a natural immunity to bird flu, and there are no immunizations available to protect us from it, so bird flu infection has the potential to reach epidemic proportions.

For a large epidemic (pandemic) to develop, three things have to happen. First, the virus must cause serious disease in people (which has occurred). Second, people must have little or no immunity to the virus and no vaccine available to protect them (again, this is true). And third, chains of infection must occur among people (lucky for us, this has not happened and might not).

WHO'S AT RISK People in all age groups have contracted and died of bird flu. The H5N1 virus strain is especially aggressive and has caused the most reported cases, primarily infecting healthy children and young adults. This is particularly alarming because influenza usually kills the very young, the very old, and the sick. However, at this point, if you are not in an area where there is an outbreak, you are probably not at risk for getting bird flu.

DEFENSIVE MEASURES According to the CDC, there is no vaccine that will protect against the H5N1 virus, but several pharmaceutical companies are working on different ones. Two common antiviral medications, amantadine (Symmetrel) and rimantadine (Flumadine), have not been effective in combating the symptoms of avian influenza, but two others, oseltamivir (Tamiflu) and zanamavir (Relenza), look promising. There is absolutely no reason to ask your physician for this medication at this point, however, even if you are traveling to affected countries.

The best defense is an easy one, and one that you will see throughout this book: Wash your hands. Frequently washing your hands with soap and hot water, especially before and after eating meals or using the bathroom, keeps a variety of bacteria and viruses at bay, including the kinds that cause bird flu. Alcohol-based sanitizers that you just rub on your hands and don't need water work well, too.

You should also get a flu shot every year. The big fear right now is that a human influenza virus and a bird flu virus could combine to form a potent virus that could easily spread among people. Flu vaccination is very successful at limiting the spread of human flu and will go a long way toward keeping this potentially deadly equation from adding up.

It's also a good idea to steer clear of wild birds; pigeons; and domesticated birds used for poultry, such as chickens, ducks, and geese, in places where there have been outbreaks among birds. These countries include Cambodia, China, Croatia, Indonesia, Japan, Kazakhstan, Korea, Malaysia, Mongolia, Romania, Russia, Thailand, Turkey, and Vietnam. You can find information about all the countries that have had cases of animal and human bird flu at the U.S. government's one-stop bird flu Web site, www.avianflu.gov.

When traveling, avoid open-air markets with live birds, and don't touch surfaces contaminated with bird droppings or feathers. And watch your children, whether abroad or at home. Children often play close to the ground and pick up all kinds of things that can harbor infections. Because many kids haven't developed good hygiene habits, they are easy prey for viruses. No evidence of transmission exists through undercooked poultry or eggs, but for any poultry-transmitted disease, precautions include:

BIOTERRORISM AGENTS: PLAGUE AND SMALLPOX

Plague:

- Caused by infection with the bacterium *Yersinia pestis*
- Occurs naturally, most often in Africa and Asia, but natural cases have been seen in the southwestern United States
- Natural cases are spread by infected rodent fleas; one type, pneumonic plague, can be spread person to person
- When weaponized, plague can be spread in an aerosolized form and cause pneumonic plague
- Can be treated with antibiotics, but no vaccine is available
- In its severe forms, plague has a mortality rate close to 100 percent when untreated; if treated, the mortality rate is 5 percent to 10 percent

Smallpox:

- Caused by infection with the variola virus
- Due to vaccination, the last natural case occurred in the 1970s, but an estimated 300 million people worldwide died from it in the twentieth century
- Easily spread from person to person
- Any occurrences of smallpox, which has been eradicated through vaccinations, would signal the use of the virus as a bioweapon
- No readily available therapy, but receiving a vaccination could lessen severity if given within four days of exposure
- Mortality rate is about 30 percent

- **Keep it cooked.** Eggshells can be contaminated with bird droppings that are full of pesky germs that can make their way into foods that use undercooked eggs. That means don't lick the beater after you make brownie batter or cookie dough, and don't eat Hollandaise sauce, homemade mayonnaise, and other foods with raw eggs as ingredients.

■ **Keep it hot.** If you're cooking chicken, turkey, or other poultry, use a meat thermometer to ensure it reaches an internal temperature of 180 degrees Fahrenheit before eating.

■ **Keep it sanitized.** When working with raw or partially cooked poultry, thoroughly wash everything that comes into contact with it. Sanitize cutting boards, knives, and other utensils by washing them in hot, soapy water, and use a disinfectant on counters and other surfaces. Wash your hands and dry them on a paper towel; cloth towels can harbor germs.

■ **Keep it separate.** If you have a pet bird, don't allow it to share food or water with other birds, especially wild ones. Keep the cage clean and wash your hands after you touch your pet.

There is speculation that other pets, such as cats, may become infected with a bird flu virus if they eat a contaminated bird, prompting some veterinarians to recommend keeping cats indoors. The close and affectionate contact between pets and owners creates a transmission risk. Although cats aren't thought to spread the virus in their feces and urine as efficiently as poultry can, be sure to wash your hands after changing the litter box.

E. coli 0157 (*Escherichia coli* 0157:H7)

CULPRIT *E. coli* is one of the many bacteria normally found in the intestines of animals, including people, and excreted in bowel movements. This particular strain (O157) is not normally found in the human intestine and poses significant risks to those who become infected by it. The bacterium can be found in the stool of cattle, especially during summer months.

INFECTION INFO Unlike other milder strains of *E. coli*, *E. coli* O157 produces a toxin that damages the intestinal lining and causes an acute disease called hemorrhagic colitis. During a bout of hemorrhagic colitis, a person experiences severe abdominal pain; diarrhea that progresses from watery to bloody; occasional vomiting; and, when the disease is at its worst, kidney failure. A high fever typically accompanies these symptoms in other infections, but it is surprisingly absent in cases of *E. coli* O157 infection. The illness runs its course in about eight days. Children are especially susceptible to *E. coli* O157 complications, which might cause kidney failure.

E. coli O157 is spread through water or food that is directly or indirectly contaminated with animal (usually cattle) feces. Unwashed fruits or vegetables, undercooked beef (especially ground beef), and unpasteurized milk are frequent vehicles for the bacterium. It also can spread person to person when people don't wash their hands often enough and through swimming in contaminated water.

WHO'S AT RISK Anyone can become infected with *E. coli* O157, but the most serious complications develop in children younger than 5 and in the elderly. In these populations, the infection can lead to hemolytic uremic syndrome, a complication that causes the kidneys to fail.

DEFENSIVE MEASURES Although undercooked hamburger has often been implicated in *E. coli* O157 outbreaks, other foods also have

BIOTERRORISM AGENTS: TULAREMIA AND VIRAL HEMORRHAGIC FEVERS

Tularemia:

- Caused by infection of the bacterium *Francisella tularensis*
- Occurs naturally in the United States (disproportionately on the island of Martha's Vineyard, which sees cases almost yearly), Europe, and Asia
- Usually spread via bug bites or exposure to infected animals (especially rabbits)
- Weaponized versions of tularemia could be spread through inhalation
- Clusters of cases would signify use as a bioweapon
- Not spread from person to person
- Can be treated with antibiotics; the U.S. Food and Drug Administration is in the process of reviewing a vaccine, but it isn't currently available
- Without treatment, mortality rate can be 30 percent to 50 percent; with prompt treatment, mortality rate is 3 percent to 5 percent

Viral Hemorrhagic Fevers (VHF):

- Many different kinds exist (including Ebola virus and Lassa fever, which occur in Africa)
- Caused by a variety of viruses
- Spread naturally in nature through infected rodents, but can spread person to person, especially when infection-control practices aren't used
- Clusters of cases where a VHF doesn't naturally occur would signify use as a bioweapon
- Most have no treatment and no available vaccine
- Mortality rates vary, but Ebola can be as high as 80 percent to 90 percent

been blamed, including alfalfa sprouts, cheese curds, unpasteurized fruit juices, dry-cured salami, lettuce, and game meat. However, any food product eaten raw or contaminated by raw meat could be infected. Outbreaks have also occurred through direct exposure to animals in petting zoos.

But before you start investing in high-power microscopes to examine all the food that comes into your kitchen, keep in mind that you can significantly cut your risk of *E. coli* O157 infection by taking a few simple precautions:

- **Soap up.** Washing your hands thoroughly and frequently helps protect you from contracting *E. coli* O157 from infected people, who may unknowingly share the bacteria. Good hand washing is especially important between family members in households where diapers are changed and toddlers need assistance after using the bathroom. If you visit a petting zoo with kids, be sure they look but don't touch and practice good hand washing.

- **Thoroughly cook ground beef.** Ground beef is a particular risk because meat from many different cows is mixed together by the ton, and it only takes a small amount of *E. coli* O157 to spoil a whole batch. Contaminated meat won't look, smell, or taste odd. Use a meat thermometer to ensure ground beef is cooked to at least 160 degrees Fahrenheit throughout. And when at a restaurant, don't hesitate to send back a pink hamburger, and ask for a new plate and bun, too.

- **Clean up after raw meat.** Wash all surfaces, counters, utensils, and cutting boards used during the preparation of raw meats, and be sure to keep raw meat separate from other ingredients.

- **Choose pasteurized products.** Avoid drinking raw (unpasteurized) milk. If *E. coli* bacteria are present on a cow's udder or on milking equipment, the bacteria could pass into raw milk supplies. Unpasteurized fruit and vegetable juices also could be contaminated with *E. coli* O157.
- **Run some water.** You should wash all raw fruits and vegetables thoroughly before eating them, but think twice about consuming even washed alfalfa sprouts. According to the CDC, the very young, the elderly, and the immunocompromised should not eat them at all because of their tendency to harbor *E. coli* O157.

Mad Cow Disease (Bovine Spongiform Encephalopathy)

CULPRIT The cause of mad cow disease is still being debated. Most authorities, however, hold that misshapen prion proteins cause the disease. These misfolded proteins are infectious when directly

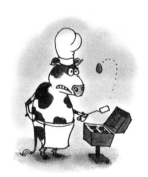

inoculated into the brain, injected into the body, or eaten. Because prions lack nucleic acid, they cannot be attacked the same way viruses are. In fact, prions are virtually indestructible.

Outbreaks of human prion disease have been caused by contaminated growth hormone produced from cadavers, from ritual cannibalism, and from eating meat from cattle with mad cow disease.

INFECTION INFO Mad cow disease is a fatal infection that causes neurological degeneration in cattle and was first noted in the

1980s. The brain wastes away and becomes spongelike, and the central nervous system is wrecked.

According to the World Health Organization, infected cattle can carry the disease for four to five years before showing symptoms. However, once symptoms appear, the degenerative disease causes death within 12 months. Signs of mad cow disease include odd changes in temperament (including extreme nervousness), weight loss, and lack of coordination. Although the exact origin of mad cow disease is unknown, it is most often transmitted to animals through manufactured high-protein feed that contains the brain or spinal cord remnants of infected animals.

A fatal brain disease in people called variant Creutzfeldt-Jakob disease (vCJD) is a result of being exposed to beef infected by mad cow disease. Like mad cow disease, vCJD causes spongelike holes in the brain and can incubate for years, but it is difficult to diagnose before it causes severe neurological damage and triggers brain deterioration; death usually occurs within a year or so. Other animals, including large felines in zoos, have acquired the infection from eating affected meat scraps.

Variant Creutzfeldt-Jakob disease is different from Creutzfeldt-Jakob disease, which was discovered more than 100 years ago. People with vCJD are usually much younger and die in 12 months to 18 months instead of four months to six months. Differences are also apparent upon microscopic examination of affected brain tissue. Variant Creutzfeldt-Jakob disease was first reported in 1996.

WHO'S AT RISK Anyone who eats beef from an animal with mad cow disease is at risk. About 150 worldwide cases of vCJD have occurred to date, nearly all associated with beef consumption in the United Kingdom. Experts are still debating whether a larger epidemic of this disease in humans will happen. Mad cow disease has also been reported to a lesser degree in other European countries, Japan, Canada, and even the United States.

DEFENSIVE MEASURES If the risk of having your brain turn to mush has you contemplating a few dietary changes, you should consider the following:

- According to the CDC, solid cuts of meat carry less risk of exposing people to the agents that cause vCJD. T-bone steak (which is a cut from near the cow's spinal column), ground beef, sausage, hot dogs, or any meat that can contain bits of brain tissue or spinal cord carry the highest risk.
- Replacing some red meats with poultry and fish, or skipping meat altogether, can reduce your risk.
- Watch what you eat when you travel. If you visit countries where mad cow disease has been reported, including the United Kingdom, skip the beef entrée.
- Milk and products made from milk are not thought to be a means of transmittal.

Cooking your hamburgers extremely well-done won't protect you, because prions aren't destroyed during any cooking process. However, your chances of running across this infection are rare because meat products cannot be imported into the United States from countries with mad cow outbreaks, and the Food and Drug Administration has stopped allowing importation of dietary supplement and cosmetic ingredients that contain bovine products from certain at-risk countries.

Necrotizing Fasciitis (Flesh-Eating Disease)

CULPRIT Group A *Streptococcus* bacteria, the same bacteria that cause strep throat, can be to blame for the bacterial infection known as the "flesh-eating" disease. However, a combination of other oxygen-using (aerobic) or oxygen-avoiding (anaerobic) bacteria can be the cause, as well.

INFECTION INFO The bacteria that cause necrotizing fasciitis can enter the body through respiratory droplets, such as those released during a sneeze or cough, or they can get in through a surgical incision or through an injury as minor as a paper cut. The bacteria multiply quickly and destroy skin and soft tissues, including the fascia, the fibrous tissue below the skin that surrounds muscle.

At its onset, necrotizing fasciitis causes flulike symptoms and severe pain in the affected area, but within a day or so, the work of the destructive bacteria becomes apparent: Swollen, dark tissue and blisters filled with black fluid develop on the infected body part. By this time, the pain disappears because the nerves are destroyed. If the disease is allowed to progress, it can cause blood pressure to drop and can send the body into shock from the toxins released by scores of bacteria. The infected person requires immediate hospitalization to receive intravenous antibiotics and to have the infected tissue surgically removed.

According to the CDC, necrotizing fasciitis kills about 20 percent of the people it afflicts, but complications due to toxic shock can push the mortality rate to 50 percent. Survivors face massive amputation, disfigured tissue, and months of skin grafts to repair damaged areas.

WHO'S AT RISK Anyone can be infected with the bacteria that cause necrotizing fasciitis. However, those with weakened immune systems, people who have diabetes, alcohol and drug abusers, the elderly, and those who undergo abdominal surgery are at increased risk.

DEFENSIVE MEASURES The best way to defend yourself against necrotizing fasciitis is to avoid the bacteria that cause it. That means washing your hands thoroughly and often, steering clear of people who have sore throat symptoms (in case they have strep throat), and taking care of injuries. If you receive a cut or abrasion, wash it thoroughly with hot water and soap and apply antibiotic ointment. And don't pop skin blisters—the National Institutes of Health says keeping the skin intact is a powerful line of defense to ward off infection.

If flesh-eating bacteria are present, you'll want to get treatment early on. Watch injured areas for signs of infection, especially if you're in a high-risk group. Look for swelling around the wound, redness, and/or drainage, and note any pain. If you have any doubts, seek medical treatment. Early intervention can save life and limb.

SARS (Severe Acute Respiratory Syndrome)

CULPRIT A newly discovered coronavirus causes SARS.

INFECTION INFO SARS is a viral respiratory illness that first appeared in China in 2002, but it soon spread to North America, South America, and Europe. It appears to have been transmitted to humans through mixing of viruses among captive animals at market in China. SARS usually spreads when an infected person coughs or sneezes, expelling droplets of fluid that come into contact with the mucous membranes (in the eyes or nose) of an uninfected person. People can also pick up SARS coronavirus by touching a surface or object contaminated by those droplets and then putting their hands to their eyes or nose.

According to the CDC, there is some suspicion among researchers that the SARS virus might spread through the air in ways that aren't yet known. The virus causes flulike symptoms, including fever, headache, muscle aches, a dry cough, and general discom-

KEEP YOUR PERSPECTIVE

Your television newscasts probably spend a good deal of time on infectious diseases, but have you heard of SLOPS? SLOPS is an acronym for severe loss of perspective syndrome. This easily treated condition is seen in a fair number of well-meaning people, particularly those who work in the news media. Those affected by SLOPS spend an amazing amount of time worrying about infections that have not involved large numbers of individuals.

For instance, according to the World Health Organization, during the SARS (severe acute respiratory syndrome) outbreak, a time period defined as November 2002 to July 2003, 8,098 people worldwide became sick with SARS that was accompanied by either pneumonia or respiratory distress syndrome, and 774 of these people died (none in the United States). Compare that to the National Highway Traffic Safety Administration's statistic that 17,105 people were killed in alcohol-related traffic crashes in the United States in 2003. Now ask yourself, which issue got more press that year? Lucky for all of us, SLOPS is the rare condition that can be cured by mind over matter.

fort. A small percentage of people with SARS may have diarrhea. Most people infected with SARS develop pneumonia.

WHO'S AT RISK Anybody can contract SARS, but health-care workers who come into contact with infected patients are most at risk. Those who are 40 and older are most likely to have complications. However, according to the CDC, SARS was not being transmitted anywhere on the globe when this book went to press.

DEFENSIVE MEASURES Although there are currently no outbreaks of SARS, there is always the chance the virus will rear its ugly head again. It's a good idea to follow basic infection-control tips. That means washing your hands well and often, or using alcohol-based hand sanitizers; covering your mouth and nose when you sneeze; not touching your nose, mouth, or eyes unless your hands are clean; and being extra vigilant in environments such as airplanes where viruses can easily jump from person to person.

West Nile Virus

CULPRIT West Nile disease is caused by the West Nile virus, which is usually spread by the *Culex* species of mosquitoes. The name comes from the area around the Nile River in Uganda, where the virus was first isolated.

INFECTION INFO Wild birds are the main source of West Nile virus. When mosquitoes feed on infected birds, they become carriers and transmit the virus to people and other animals. The West Nile virus enters the bloodstream through a mosquito bite, then multiplies and spreads and can eventually make its way to the brain, where it causes inflammation. In very rare cases, West Nile virus has been transmitted from mother to baby during pregnancy, through breast milk, and through organ transplants and blood transfusions from an infected donor. West Nile virus does not otherwise spread from person to person.

Only a very small percentage of mosquitoes are actually infected with West Nile virus, and not everyone bitten by an infected mosquito will become sick. The good news is if illness does occur, the body can usually fight it off, and many people will have no symptoms. In those who do develop a more severe form of illness, the symptoms of fever, headache, muscle aches, swollen glands, and joint pain subside within several days. In rare cases, West Nile virus can cause encephalitis (inflammation of the brain) and meningitis (inflammation of the membranes that surround the brain and spinal cord). No preventive vaccine is available for West Nile virus.

WHO'S AT RISK Anyone who comes into contact with infected mosquitoes can contract West Nile virus, but people 50 and older or those who have weakened immune systems are most at risk for complications. West Nile virus has been found in all lower 48 states, but those who live in warmer climates are more likely to encounter infected mosquitoes. People who work outdoors also have a greater chance of being bitten by an infected mosquito. Many state health department Web sites have information about West Nile prevalence within their borders.

DEFENSIVE MEASURES To keep West Nile virus away, you need to keep mosquitoes away. Wearing insect repellent is just one of the many things you can do to protect yourself from West Nile virus:

■ **Buy the right bug spray.** When you reach for a can of insect repellent, be sure it includes oil of lemon eucalyptus or chemicals such as picaridin, permethrin, or DEET. DEET is toxic, so it should be applied sparingly to the skin. Don't apply a repellent that is more than 30 percent DEET on children, and never put it on their hands.

■ **Wear a layer of protection.** When outside in heavy mosquito areas, wear long sleeves, long pants, and socks. Mosquitoes can bite through thin fabrics, so spray clothing with insect repellent.

■ **Steer clear of standing water.** Standing water, whether in a puddle, a wading pool, a birdbath, clogged gutters, or a tire swing, is the mosquito's version of a hot nightclub. Get rid of the water and you get rid of the mosquito breeding ground.

■ **Shield the stroller.** If you are taking your baby on a walk, use a mosquito net. There are many types available for nearly any make and model of stroller or carriage.

■ **Watch the time.** If you are outdoors in the early morning or early evening, you're more likely to get bitten because more mosquitoes will be buzzing around.

■ **Keep the outside out.** Check the screens on your home's windows and doors. If they're in good shape, mosquitoes won't be moving in.

■ **Make the call.** If you come across a dead bird, call your local health authorities. Whatever you do, don't touch it with your bare hands. It's important to keep a firm handle on West Nile virus activity even before it affects humans, and the information you provide can alert authorities to the need for better mosquito control.

■ **Put away your credit card.** Ignore those infomercials about "ultrasonic" mosquito devices or cases of vitamin B. The CDC says these aren't effective in preventing mosquito bites.

Chapter 2   Old Friends

Bird flu and mad cow disease may be getting most of the media attention these days, but old infectious stalwarts—the common cold, the flu, and pneumonia—do far more damage every year. These common illnesses are frustrating at best, deadly at their worst. But even though we have no cures for these familiar foes, you can protect yourself from them.

Common Cold

CULPRIT Take your pick: More than 200 viruses could be responsible for your cold. About 35 percent of those viruses belong to the rhinovirus family.

INFECTION INFO You wake up with the sniffles and a mild headache, and by lunch your throat begins to hurt and your nose starts flowing. By the time you make it home for dinner, you have a low fever, a cough, and tissues stuffed up your nostrils. Your miserable situation is thanks to a friendly, neighborhood cold virus.

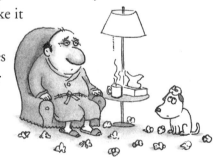

Cold viruses love the warm, moist environment of your nose and upper respiratory tract, which is where they grow and wreak their havoc. Cold viruses travel to the nasal passages by different routes. Some enter via airborne droplets when an infected person coughs or sneezes, and some are carried on hands and common objects, such as phones, drinking glasses, and toys. Once you get the viral particles on your hands, all you need to do is touch your nose, mouth (which is part of your upper respiratory tract), or eyes (the eyes drain into the nasal passages), and the virus has found a new temporary home.

After you've been exposed to a cold virus, symptoms will show up in two or three days, and you should be over the worst of your sniffles and coughing in a week or two. Most people will overcome a cold without complications, but the occasional cold sufferer might end up with a sinus infection (sinusitis, see page 83) or an ear infection—both of which might require a round of antibiotics.

Cold season lasts from early fall to early spring and hits its peak during the cold, dry winter months. People spend most of their time indoors when it's cold, making it easy for viruses to jump from host to host. Once you have a cold, you'll do well to follow Mom's instructions—get lots of rest, drink plenty of fluids, and eat some chicken soup (the steam helps your stuffy nose and chest). You can also treat your symptoms with over-the-counter cold medicines, but be aware these are not cures and will do nothing to shorten the duration of your cold.

WHO'S AT RISK Everyone is at risk of catching a cold. Adults get about two to four colds every year, and children get eight to ten annually. For Americans, that adds up to about two billion colds a year. The good news is once you get one particular cold virus, you develop immunity to that strain for life. So by the time you hit 60, if you're in the norm, you'll average only one cold every year.

DEFENSIVE MEASURES There is no cure for the common cold, but you can protect yourself from as many sneezes as possible by:

■ **Washing your hands.** Your best protection against a cold virus is to wash your hands often with soap and water. Be extra vigilant with hand washing during cold season if you work with kids or if you are around someone with a cold, especially someone in your own household.

■ **Keeping a stash of gel.** If you can't always get to a sink, the Centers for Disease Control and Prevention (CDC) recommends keeping some alcohol-based gel cleanser with you and using it often.

■ **Keeping your hands away from your face.** Because cold viruses like to get into your body through your mouth, nose, and eyes, keeping your hands away from these body parts is essential to keeping colds at bay.

■ **Using your own stuff.** Don't use a cold-sufferer's phone, keyboard, pen, drinking glass, or any other item where a cold virus can lie in wait.

■ **Doing some disinfecting.** Viruses are hardy creatures that can live up to three hours on objects. Use a disinfectant that specifically targets cold viruses to clean common areas.

■ **Keeping that immune system humming.** Eat right, exercise, and manage stress to keep your immune system at its best to help you fight off any cold bug.

■ **Avoiding the crowd.** Because cold viruses are so contagious, you improve your chances of not getting one if you stay away from the pack.

■ **Being wary of popular "cures."** There is no conclusive scientific evidence that echinacea, zinc, or vitamin C can cure a

FEED A COLD AND STARVE A FEVER?

This bit of folk wisdom has been bouncing around for centuries. The advice may have evolved from the idea that illnesses could be classified as either low-temperature conditions (such as the common "cold") or high-temperature conditions (those causing fever). To combat a cold condition, it sounds reasonable to feed a person's internal fireplace with food. The logic then follows that when an illness raises the body's temperature, cutting back on the "fuel" should help.

However, scientific evidence does not support this advice; many illnesses must simply run their course regardless of your food intake. Nevertheless, if you are stuck in bed with a cold and a loved one brings over your favorite healthful foods, it is still okay to chow down. Alternatively, you may lose your appetite while fighting a febrile (fever-based) sickness. It's okay to miss a meal or two as long as you are keeping up your fluid intake.

cold. In fact, taking too much of one of these can cause unwanted side effects, such as nausea.

Influenza (Flu)

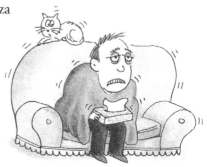

CULPRIT Three types of influenza viruses, influenza A, B, and C, cause "the flu." Type A viruses cause the most problems—they are responsible for worldwide influenza pandemics. Type B influenza viruses cause smaller outbreaks, and type C viruses (which are much less common) cause mild symptoms. The A and B types of viruses are constantly changing, while C viruses are fairly stable.

INFECTION INFO An influenza virus is spread much like a cold virus; you can get one either by inhaling an airborne droplet from an infected person's cough or sneeze or by touching something (doorknob, computer keyboard, phone, eating utensil, etc.) that has an influenza virus on it (one can live for several hours on an inanimate object). And because infected people are contagious for a day or two before showing any symptoms, many carriers are completely unaware they are sharing an influenza virus. What makes this infection such a big deal? According to the CDC, the flu kills 36,000 people in the United States every year. The deaths are primarily in the elderly or those who have underlying heart, lung, liver, or kidney disease.

You'll develop symptoms within 72 hours of being exposed to an influenza virus. Although symptoms can mimic a bad cold, there are some definite differences. Classic signs that you have the flu are those notorious muscle aches; a fever, which usually ranges from 101 degrees to 103 degrees Fahrenheit in adults and higher in children; chills; a dry cough; and extreme fatigue. These symptoms will accompany coldlike problems, such as a runny and stuffy nose, a headache, and a sore throat. Some people with the flu might experience vomiting and nausea. It usually takes a week to ten days to fully recover.

Because the flu is a virus, it can't be treated with antibiotics, but there are some prescription antiviral drugs that can shorten the time you're sick. You can also treat your symptoms with over-the-counter medicines such as acetaminophen and cough sup-pressants. (Avoid giving aspirin to children because of the possi-ble risk of Reye's syndrome.) The flu can lead to more serious illnesses, like pneumonia, so if you start experiencing troubling symptoms that get worse after you start feeling better, be sure to tell your physician.

WHO'S AT RISK Anyone can get the flu, but those most at risk of having complications are the elderly, young children (especially those 6 months old to 23 months old), pregnant women, people who have chronic heart or lung conditions or other serious dis-eases, and those who have weakened immune systems.

HAND WASHING: "THE WHEN"

You've probably seen the signs in restaurant bathrooms that say, "Employees must wash hands before returning to work." This is an excellent idea, but *everyone* should wash their hands after using the bathroom, whether in a restaurant, at home, or anywhere else. Hand washing is the single most important way to prevent the spread of infection.

You should wash your hands:

- Before touching any kind of food
- Before treating a wound
- After using the bathroom or changing a baby's diaper
- After touching pets or cleaning their environment
- After sneezing, coughing, or blowing your nose
- After touching raw meat, poultry, or fish
- After working in the yard
- After caring for an ill person
- After handling garbage

DEFENSIVE MEASURES The best way you can protect yourself from the flu is to get a vaccination every year. Influenza viruses are constantly changing, so the strain of virus you were protected against last year is not likely the same strain striking this year. Get a flu shot at the very beginning of flu season (in October or November) so your immunity peaks when influenza outbreaks do (generally late December to mid-March). However, even getting vaccinated in December or January will provide some protection. Flu shots are highly recommended for people who are at high risk of contracting influenza or of having severe complications. Talk with your physician if you think you fall into one of these groups. Anti-influenza medications, such as amantadine (Symmetrel), rimantidine (Flumadine), and oseltamavir (Tamiflu) can also be used to prevent and treat the infection.

In addition to getting an influenza vaccination, you should follow the preventive tips outlined in the common cold profile.

Pneumonia

CULPRIT Pneumonia has many causes—viruses, bacteria (most commonly *Streptococcus pneumoniae*), mycoplasmas (disease-spreading bacteria that are smaller than, and lack the cell walls of, typical bacteria), fungi, and even certain chemicals. According to the American Lung Association, viruses are to blame for half of all pneumonia cases.

INFECTION INFO Pneumonia is an infection that settles in one or both lungs. The lung tissue becomes inflamed and the microscopic air sacs fill with fluid. The combination of swelling and

fluid can hinder the movement of oxygen into the bloodstream.
Symptoms vary from mild to serious depending on the type of
pneumonia contracted, but basic symp-
toms include an intense cough, fever,
chills, and fatigue. Some types of
pneumonia mimic a cold and
include muscle aches, sore
throat, and a headache. In more
serious cases, pneumonia can
cause chest pain, a racing pulse,
and breathlessness.

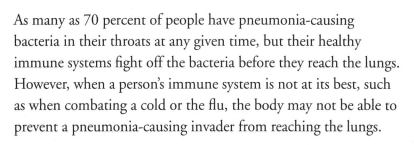

As many as 70 percent of people have pneumonia-causing
bacteria in their throats at any given time, but their healthy
immune systems fight off the bacteria before they reach the lungs.
However, when a person's immune system is not at its best, such
as when combating a cold or the flu, the body may not be able to
prevent a pneumonia-causing invader from reaching the lungs.

Viruses usually cause milder forms of pneumonia than bacteria
do. A viral pneumonia will make you feel icky, but it should
clear up on its own within a week or two. However, because
pneumonia affects your lungs, no case should be ignored. The
best course of action is the same as for the flu—get plenty of rest,
drink fluids, and take steamy showers to loosen up the gunk in
your lungs. You can also manage your fever, aches and pains, and
cough with over-the-counter medicines. Bacterial pneumonias
can be much more serious and can lead to long-term complications, but fortunately, they usually can be successfully treated
with antibiotics.

No matter the cause, pneumonia is a serious infection, even with prompt medical treatment. According to the CDC's National Center for Health Statistics, pneumonia killed almost 65,000 people in the United States in 2002 (the last year for which statistics were available).

WHO'S AT RISK People with weaker-than-normal immune systems are at greatest risk of contracting pneumonia. This includes children younger than 2 years; those 65 and older; and people with chronic health conditions, such as lung or heart disease, sickle cell anemia, or diabetes. People fighting cancer or AIDS are also at high risk. Hospitalized people, especially those in an intensive care unit and/or on a ventilator, and those who live in nursing homes are at a much greater risk for developing hospital-acquired pneumonia. Smokers are also more susceptible to developing pneumonia.

HAND WASHING: "THE HOW"

Just because you can't see any dirt or grime doesn't mean your hands are clean. Germs are invisible, so follow this method to get your hands as clean as possible:

1. Wet your hands in warm, running water.
2. Apply liquid soap or a clean bar of soap.
3. Lather well.
4. Rub hands vigorously for at least 15 seconds.
5. Scrub your wrists, the back of your hands, between your fingers, and under your fingernails.
6. Rinse well.
7. Dry hands with a clean or disposable towel.
8. Use the towel to turn off the faucet.

DEFENSIVE MEASURES Maintaining a healthy lifestyle is the best way to prevent pneumonia. That includes getting a flu vaccination each year, because the flu is a common precursor to pneumonia, as well as not smoking, eating a healthy diet, and getting plenty of exercise and rest. These actions will boost your immune system and keep your cold or flu from turning into something much more serious.

There is a vaccine available that fights off the bacteria-based pneumococcal pneumonia. This vaccine is effective in 80 percent of healthy adults and certainly helps high-risk groups lower their odds of developing pneumonia. If you are at high risk, or if you have a baby younger than 23 months, you should speak with your physician about this vaccine and the new pneumococcal vaccine for young children.

Chapter 3 — Getting Your Baby Shots

Children are born with temporary protection from many diseases, thanks to antibodies from the mother passed through the placenta. Within a year, however, this defense is lost and a number of illnesses come knocking at the door. Childhood vaccinations protect us from these diseases, but when they aren't complete, the bugs come crawling back.

Chickenpox (Varicella)

CULPRIT The varicella-zoster virus, a member of the herpesvirus family, causes chickenpox. The virus is spread through the air when someone who has it coughs or sneezes, spreading viral particles that are then inhaled by a nonimmune person. Contact with the fluid of chickenpox blisters can also spread the virus, but it does not live long on inanimate objects, such as doorknobs.

INFECTION INFO Chickenpox causes a remarkably itchy skin rash that is easy to identify because of its small red bumps that look like insect bites or pimples. The bumps first appear on the back, face, scalp, and abdomen, and then can spread nearly everywhere else, including the mouth, nose, ears, and genitals, but they are concentrated on the face and body. The bumps develop into blisters that are filled with clear fluid that later turns cloudy. These blisters break and develop into open sores and then dry brown scabs. All stages of the lesions can be present at the same time. Chickenpox usually lasts about seven days in children but several days longer in adults.

WHO'S AT RISK Before the chickenpox vaccine was available, children younger than 15 were the particular risk group, but anyone could be infected. Chickenpox is usually a mild illness, but complications, such as viral pneumonia, inflammation of the brain (encephalitis), and, more commonly, bacterial infection of the skin can occur. Anyone who experiences chickenpox as a child is at risk for shingles later in life (see the shingles profile later in this chapter for more information).

DEFENSIVE MEASURES Chickenpox is very contagious, but immunization with the varicella vaccine is an effective weapon against it. Beyond that, avoid contact with anyone who has chickenpox. If contact is unavoidable, wash hands and disinfect surfaces, particularly when dealing with the fluid-filled blisters.

The varicella vaccine has been administered since 1995 and is one of the routine immunizations given to children between 12 months and 18 months of age. The vaccine is more than 95 percent effective in preventing the severest form of the virus and is 80 percent to 90 percent effective at preventing milder forms of the infection. Children who develop chickenpox after being vaccinated will experience a weaker form of the disease.

Older children and adolescents who haven't received the vaccine, and who have not had chickenpox, should be immunized. However, instead of a single vaccine dose, adolescents 12 and older require two doses given a minimum of four weeks apart.

REYE'S SYNDROME

Reye's syndrome can affect the blood, liver, and brain of children and teenagers who are recovering from a viral infection (such as chickenpox or influenza). Although there is no conclusive proof, using aspirin to treat a viral disease appears to be linked to the incidence of Reye's syndrome. The rare syndrome, which is still not well understood, usually appears within a week after the onset of a viral illness.

Symptoms of Reye's syndrome are continual vomiting and nausea, lethargy, indifference, irrational behavior or delirium, and rapid breathing. In the later stages, breathing becomes sluggish and the child can become unconscious or comatose. The liver might be enlarged, but there is usually no jaundice or fever.

The duration varies, as does the severity. Reye's syndrome can be mild and self-limiting, or in rare cases, it can progress to death in a matter of hours. The progression can stop at any stage, and complete recovery is usually seen in five to ten days.

The viral illnesses that lead to Reye's syndrome are contagious, but the syndrome itself is not. Contact your physician if you suspect Reye's syndrome in your child or if you have questions about which medications are safe.

It's also important to watch the calendar. Chickenpox occurs most often in late winter and early spring. An infected person is contagious two days before the rash appears and until all the blisters have formed scabs. A child with chickenpox should be kept out of school or day care until all the blisters have dried, which is usually about one week.

Susceptible pregnant women should steer clear of a person with chickenpox. If a pregnant woman who isn't immune gets the disease, her baby has a small risk of birth defects, and the mother has a higher risk of developing serious complications, such as varicella pneumonia.

Newborns born to women who develop chickenpox right before or right after delivery can develop life-threatening varicella. These infants can get some protection from varicella-zoster immune globulin (VZIG). VZIG also can be given to high-risk children, such as those with leukemia or those taking immune-suppressing drugs. Never give aspirin to a child who gets chicken-pox because of the risk of Reye's syndrome, a rare, but potentially deadly, disease.

Healthy children who have had chickenpox don't need to be vaccinated; they are usually immune to the disease for life.

Diphtheria

CULPRIT Diphtheria is caused by infection with the bacterium *Corynebacterium diphtheriae,* which spreads easily and quickly.

INFECTION INFO Diphtheria mainly affects the nose and throat. In its early stages, people may mistake diphtheria for a severe sore throat accompanied by a low-grade fever and swollen neck glands. The *C. diphtheriae* bacterium creates a toxin that can lead to a thick coating in the nose, throat, or airway. This coating is easy to spot because of its unusual gray or black color. The toxin affects the throat and neck, as well as the heart and nervous system, and can cause:

- A swollen neck (the "bull neck")
- Breathing problems and swallowing difficulties
- Slurred speech
- Double vision
- Disorders of the heart rhythm
- Shock (rapid heartbeat and clammy, cold, and pale skin)

Even with proper treatment, diphtheria kills about 10 percent of those who contract it. Treatment with antibiotics and antitoxins often takes place in a hospital, and a ventilator may be needed to facilitate breathing.

WHO'S AT RISK Children 5 and younger are especially at risk for getting diphtheria with severe complications. Children who are malnourished, who live in crowded or unsanitary conditions, or who have not been immunized have an even greater risk.

DEFENSIVE MEASURES Preventing diphtheria means immunizing your child with the diphtheria/tetanus/pertussis (DTP or DTaP) vaccine. Most cases of diphtheria occur in people who haven't received the vaccine or who haven't received the entire course of it. The disease is rarely diagnosed in the United States, but it occurs more frequently in developing countries.

The DTP or DTaP vaccine is given at 2, 4, and 6 months of age, with a booster given at 12 to 18 months of age and another when the child is between 4 and 6 years old. Booster shots should be given every ten years after age 6 to maintain protection. The amount of diphtheria toxoid (inactivated toxin) in the adult vaccine (Td vaccine) is lower.

Those infected by *C. diphtheriae* can transmit it to others for up to four weeks, even if they don't have any symptoms. Diphtheria is a highly contagious disease, so anyone who has it must be isolated to prevent its spread.

Because diphtheria is easily contracted through sneezing, coughing, laughing, or even sharing a drinking glass or toy, it's important to remain vigilant about hand washing, especially when children are sharing things. Sanitizing surfaces, utensils, and other items with hot water and soap or a bleach-based cleaner is essential.

If you're not sure if your child has been vaccinated against diphtheria, speak with your physician. You should also be sure your own booster immunizations are current. International studies have shown that a significant percentage of adults older than 40 aren't adequately protected against diphtheria.

German Measles (Rubella)

CULPRIT German measles is caused by the rubella virus.

INFECTION INFO The rubella virus spreads easily through coughing and sneezing, but the disease is generally mild. In fact, it is sometimes called the "three-day measles." Symptoms include a red rash, headache, loss of appetite, mild conjunctivitis (inflammation of the lining of the eyelids), swollen lymph nodes (especially in front of the ear), joint pain and swelling, and a stuffy or runny nose, but many people who are infected experience no symptoms.

The rubella virus can pass through the bloodstream of a pregnant woman to her developing child. When this happens, particularly in early stages of pregnancy, the rubella virus can cause mental retardation, deafness, cataracts, and other congenital defects that are collectively known as congenital rubella syndrome (CRS). An infant who has CRS can shed the virus in body fluids for a year or more and can pass the virus to people who have not been immunized. Thanks to immunization, German measles and CRS cases in the United States are rare.

WHO'S AT RISK Children ages 5 to 9 who have not been immunized are at risk, as are developing babies of infected pregnant women. Nonimmunized young adults are also in danger of contracting German measles.

DEFENSIVE MEASURES Rubella is preventable with vaccination. If you're planning a pregnancy, be sure your immunizations are

WHAT IS AN ANTIBIOTIC?

You may see the words antimicrobial and antibiotic used interchangeably, but they are not the same thing.

An antimicrobial agent is any natural or synthetic chemical that kills or inhibits the growth of a bacterium, fungus, or virus. An antibiotic is a compound created by a natural microorganism that kills or inhibits bacteria only. All antibiotics are antimicrobials, but not all antimicrobials are antibiotics.

Alexander Fleming discovered the value of antibiotics in 1928, when he observed that the mold *Penicillium notatum* inhibited colonies of the bacterium *Staphylococcus aureus*, proving that the fungus produced an antibacterial agent. However, penicillin use in the medical field did not begin until the 1940s, when Howard Florey and Ernst Chain isolated the active ingredient.

current. If you already are or may be pregnant, you'll have to wait until after your child is delivered before receiving the vaccination. (You must protect yourself from pregnancy for at least four weeks after being immunized.) You also should avoid contact with anyone infected by the rubella virus, but because infected people don't always have symptoms, this can be difficult.

The rubella vaccine is usually given to babies at 12 to 15 months of age as part of the measles/mumps/rubella (MMR) immunization. A second dose is given at 4 to 6 years of age.

Invasive H. Flu
(Haemophilus Influenzae Type b, Hib Disease)

CULPRIT This infection is caused by the *Haemophilus influenzae* type b (Hib) bacterium, which is spread through discharge from the throat or nose of an infected person, either by coughing, sneezing, or speaking at close range. Although initially thought to be the cause of influenza, Hib disease is not related to any form of influenza virus.

INFECTION INFO Invasive H. flu can cause bacterial meningitis, a potentially fatal brain infection, or other serious, often deadly, infections in children. However, with the development and widespread use of effective Hib vaccines, few cases are now diagnosed in the developed world. A person does not have to have symptoms to spread the infection. Besides meningitis, invasive H. flu infection can cause pneumonia; epiglottitis (severe swelling above the voice box that makes breathing difficult); and infections of the blood, joints, bones, and pericardium (the covering of the heart). In kids, less severe infections can include, but are not limited to, middle ear infection, conjunctivitis, and sinus infection.

WHO'S AT RISK Without immunization, children 5 years of age and younger are at risk, and invasive H. flu occurs most often in children ages 3 months to 2 years. As children grow older, they are less likely to develop the disease—few cases occur after age 5.

DEFENSIVE MEASURES The most effective prevention is the invasive H. flu (Hib) vaccine, which should be given to your child at 2 months of age, 4 months of age, 6 months of age (depending on the type of vaccine), and 12 to 15 months of age (be sure to ask which vaccine schedule your child's shots should follow). You also should prevent contact with children known to be infected with invasive H. flu. If your child is exposed to the infection, he or she can be given rifampin (Rifadin, Rimactane), an antibiotic that is active against the invasive H. flu bacterium.

Measles (Rubeola)

CULPRIT A highly contagious virus is to blame for measles. The infection spreads through airborne droplets when someone who is infected with the virus sneezes or coughs.

INFECTION INFO Measles is a respiratory infection that can have deadly consequences. The first symptoms of the disease mimic the common cold: runny nose, hacking cough, and red watery eyes. However, measles also causes a fever and a skin rash of red or brownish-red blotches that start at the forehead and spread downward to cover the body. Koplik's spots, which are tiny red spots with white centers that appear inside the mouth, also indicate the presence of measles. Because a virus causes measles, antibiotics are not effective. The virus must run its course, which takes about two weeks.

Complications of measles can include brain infection and pneumonia. However, these occur more commonly in malnourished or immune-deficient people.

WHO'S AT RISK Children who have not been immunized against measles are at greatest risk. Your child's chance of contracting measles is very slight if he or she has been properly vaccinated.

DEFENSIVE MEASURES Stick to your physician- or state-recommended vaccination schedule for the best protection against measles. The

MONKEYPOX ON THE PRAIRIE

Monkeypox is an uncommon viral infection that occurs naturally in parts of Central and West Africa. Although monkeypox occurs in monkeys and can infect humans, the virus's natural hosts are a variety of African rodents. The infection causes a fever, swollen lymph glands, and a rash with fluid-filled pockets (called vesicles) in people, but it is rarely fatal.

There had never been an outbreak of monkeypox in the United States until June 2003, when cases appeared in the Midwest. The outbreak was traced to the importation of Gambian giant pouched rats, one or several of which had the monkeypox virus. At some point, the rats were kept close to a number of prairie dogs that were eventually sold in pet stores and at pet swap meets. Dozens of children and adults contracted monkeypox from infected prairie dogs; all recovered.

live weakened measles virus vaccine (the only type currently available) is part of routine MMR immunizations that are given at 12 to 15 months of age and 4 to 6 years of age.

Infants are typically protected from measles for six to eight months after birth, thanks to immunity passed on from the mother. However, if there is a measles outbreak or if you will be taking your infant to an area of the world where measles is still prevalent, the vaccine can be given at 9 months of age, but this shot should still be followed by the regularly scheduled MMR vaccinations when the child is 12 to 15 months old and 4 to 6 years old.

If someone in your immediate family has measles, chances are good that your unvaccinated child will get it, too. Isolation is the key to prevention in such cases, as is following your physician's recommendations. In most cases, you or your child can take acetaminophen or nonsteroidal anti-inflammatory drugs (NSAIDs) to treat the fever that accompanies measles, but children shouldn't take aspirin because of the risk of Reye's syndrome.

Mumps

CULPRIT Mumps is caused by a virus that is spread through nose and mouth fluids, particularly via sneezing, coughing, or laughing. Children can easily transmit mumps when sharing items such as toys, cups, and crayons.

INFECTION INFO Mumps primarily affects the saliva-producing parotid glands. These are found at the back of each cheek between the ear and jaw, and at least one side will swell remarkably due to mumps. Swallowing, talking, chewing, or drinking acidic beverages (such as orange juice) can be excruciating.

Mumps begins with a high fever, a headache, and a loss of appetite. It takes one week for the cheek swelling to go down and a total of ten to 12 days to fully recover. In rare cases, mumps can lead to

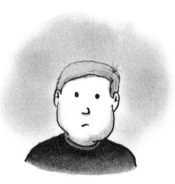

swelling of the brain or other organs. Adolescent boys and adult men can also develop an inflammation of the testicles known as orchitis (however, sterility is rare because only one testicle is usually involved). Because mumps is a viral infection, antibiotics have no effect, so you just have to manage the pain and let the virus work itself out.

WHO'S AT RISK Most cases of mumps are in children ages 5 to 14, but the number of young adults infected has been slowly rising during the past 20 years. Children 12 months and younger are usually not infected.

DEFENSIVE MEASURES The best way to prevent mumps is to be immunized. You can receive the mumps vaccine alone or, as is more common, as part of the MMR immunization.

Like many viral infections, mumps spreads easily from person to person, especially among children. Keep your kid healthy by:

- Teaching your child good hand-washing habits.
- Choosing a child care provider with exemplary sanitation practices. Questions to ask include: Are children allowed to

share toys without a disinfection process? Is play equipment wiped down with antimicrobial cleansers?

■ Understanding the "sick child" policies at your child's day care or school. Does having a high fever mean a child can't attend? If not, maybe it should.

Nevertheless, because mumps is contagious two days before symptoms begin, and because mumps can be spread from people who are infected but show no symptoms, immunization is still the best defense.

Polio (Infantile Paralysis, Poliomyelitis)

CULPRIT Polio is caused by a virus that enters the body through the mouth, usually from hands contaminated with the stool of an infected person. Objects touched by contaminated hands, such as eating utensils, can also spread the virus. There are three types of poliovirus, so a person could possibly be infected three times.

INFECTION INFO In about 95 percent of cases, polio produces no symptoms at all (known as asymptomatic polio). In the 4 percent to 8 percent of cases in which there are symptoms (symptomatic polio), the illness appears in three forms:

■ Abortive polio is limited to flulike symptoms, such as upper respiratory infection, fever, sore throat, and a general feeling of illness.

■ Nonparalytic polio is a more serious form and produces symptoms of mild meningitis, such as sensitivity to light and neck stiffness.

■ Paralytic polio is a severe, debilitating form of the disease that occurs in about 1 percent to 2 percent of cases. It can result in partial or full paralysis of the breathing muscles and extremities, necessitating breathing support—in fact, the "iron lung" was developed for people with paralytic polio.

WHO'S AT RISK Polio is most common in infants and young children, but severe complications have occurred most often in adults. Although cases of polio are basically nonexistent in the United States today, the disease is still a big problem in some developing countries.

DEFENSIVE MEASURES There hasn't been a polio epidemic in the United States since the 1950s, but the need for protection from the virus remains. The two most effective ways to prevent polio are:

■ **Cleanliness.** Polio is transmitted primarily through ingesting items, directly or indirectly, that are contaminated with feces. Not all stools carry the virus, but it's a good idea to wash hands after using the bathroom, changing a diaper, or coming into contact with questionable materials.

■ **Immunization.** The inactivated polio vaccine (IPV) used today in the United States stimulates the immune system to produce antibodies that fight the polio virus if a person comes in contact with it. Dr. Jonas Salk developed the first IPV in 1955, and an enhanced-potency version came about in 1988. Other parts of the world use an oral polio vaccine (OPV) that was first developed by Dr. Albert Sabin in 1961. OPV is based on a live, but weakened, form of the virus. OPV is cheaper, doesn't have to be administered by health-care professionals, and unlike IPV is effective in stopping outbreaks of the "wild" poliovirus (those outbreaks not related to the vaccine). However, it can, on rare occasions, cause paralysis.

In the United States, it's currently recommended that children have four doses of IPV between the ages of 2 months and 6 years. The Centers for Disease Control and Prevention and the American Academy of Pediatrics recommend three equally spaced doses of IPV be given before the age of 18 months, plus an IPV booster given between the ages of 4 and 6, when children are entering school.

If you're planning to travel outside the United States, particularly to countries where polio still exists, be sure that you and your family are up to date on complete polio vaccinations.

MEET THE EPIDEMIOLOGIST

An epidemiologist is a scientist who studies the factors that contribute to the occurrence or absence of a disease in a population. Although they are mostly interested in the study of diseases that relate to people, some epidemiologists follow diseases in animals and plants. Epidemiologists, as their title implies, determine whether a disease is epidemic in a population. An epidemic occurs when the number of cases of an illness in a community or region exceeds the disease's endemic rate, or the normal number of cases. If the epidemic spreads to much of the world, it is referred to as a pandemic.

Epidemiologists are important people in science, and their work is fascinating. It's so intriguing that a November 2001 *New Yorker* cartoon by William Hamilton pictured a high-brow party with a guest telling the host, "And it was so typically brilliant of you to have invited an epidemiologist."

Afghanistan, India, Nigeria, and Pakistan still have endemic polio circulating, and the virus could be introduced to other countries. If the polio virus were to occur in a country where not enough people have been immunized, it would spread like wildfire.

Shingles (Herpes Zoster)

CULPRIT Shingles is caused by the varicella-zoster virus, the same virus that causes chickenpox. After a chickenpox infection, the virus can lie dormant in nerve cells and may later reactivate, affect nerves just under the skin, and produce a tingling, itching, painful, and often bandlike rash known as shingles. As many as 10 percent to 20 percent of adults who had chickenpox as children will develop shingles.

INFECTION INFO Shingles is characterized by clustered red bumps that appear on one side of the body or face. It takes seven to ten days for the virus to run its course, during which time the itchy, painful bumps turn into blisters and crust over. You may see changes in the color of the skin when the scabs fall off. In bad cases of shingles, these color changes last a lifetime. The pain of shingles can linger for one to three months or longer, a condition called postherpetic neuralgia. If shingles occurs in the eye area, it can cause swollen eyelids, redness, pain, and can affect vision—in rare cases, it can cause serious vision problems.

Shingles isn't contagious, but the varicella-zoster virus is, so someone infected with shingles can transmit chickenpox, not shingles, to others who aren't immune to the virus.

WHO'S AT RISK Adults 50 and older and people with weakened immune systems are primarily at risk. Shingles is rare in children and usually takes a milder form. Only people who have had chickenpox can develop shingles.

DEFENSIVE MEASURES In children who have received the chickenpox vaccination, breakthrough chickenpox infections—usually quite mild—might occur. Scientific observations of vaccinated children have found that some will develop shingles at a later point in life. This is usually due to silent infection with the natural virus and not the weakened vaccine strain.

In May 2006, the Food and Drug Administration approved a new variant of the chickenpox vaccine that was designed to prevent shingles or make any subsequent shingles episodes milder. This new and more potent version of the chickenpox vaccine boosts immunity but is only for adults 60 and older.

Tetanus (Lockjaw)

CULPRIT Tetanus is caused by a toxin produced by a bacterium called *Clostridium tetani.* Spores (reproductive cells) of *C. tetani* are found in soil and enter the body through a skin wound. Once the germinating spores develop into mature bacteria, the bacteria produce a tetanospasmin, a neurotoxin (a protein that acts as a poison to the body's nervous system) that causes muscle spasms.

INFECTION INFO In the developed world, tetanus is a rare, but serious, illness. It often begins with muscle spasms in the jaw, called trismus, or "lockjaw." These spasms are accompanied by difficulty swallowing and painful stiffness in the muscles of the neck, shoulders, or back. These spasms can spread to the muscles of the abdomen, upper arms, and thighs. If diagnosed and treated early, recovery is possible but takes several weeks.

Keep in mind that stepping on a rusty nail is not the only way to contract tetanus. Skin punctures from nonsterile needles, such as those used for tattooing or piercing, can cause tetanus. Remember, too, that even if the instrument or wound site *looks* clean, it can still be contaminated.

Another form of tetanus, neonatal tetanus, occurs in newborns who are delivered in unsanitary conditions, especially if the umbilical cord stump becomes contaminated. This is very rare in the United States.

FEVER FALSEHOOD

Myth: All fevers must be treated with fever medication.

Fact: Fevers require treatment only if they cause discomfort, but most don't until they go above 102 degrees Fahrenheit.

WHO'S AT RISK Tetanus cannot be spread from person to person—it occurs after the tetanus-causing bacterial spores enter the body. Children who have not received the full schedule of DTP or DTaP vaccines and adults who have not had a booster in ten years are at risk. Newborns who are born to unimmunized mothers in unsanitary conditions are also at risk of getting tetanus.

DEFENSIVE MEASURES The prevention of tetanus is a relatively simple task. First, clean all wounds and remove any foreign material or dead tissue. Tetanus bacteria are strict anaerobes—that is, they only grow in the absence of oxygen—so good wound care is very important.

However, because it can be difficult even for medical professionals to completely clean out a puncture wound, you must also be sure your child receives routine tetanus vaccinations. The DTP or DTaP vaccine is given at 2, 4, and 6 months of age, with a booster given at 12 to 18 months and another when the child is between 4 and 6 years old. After that, a tetanus and diphtheria booster (Td) is recommended at 11 to 12 years of age, and then every ten years through adulthood.

If you or your child have been previously immunized but are injured in a way that increases tetanus risk (such as stepping on a rusty nail or cutting your hand with a knife), a booster shot may be necessary if it's been several years since the last one. This shot is known as postexposure tetanus prophylaxis.

Neonatal tetanus can be prevented when a pregnant woman receives tetanus immunizations and delivers her baby in sanitary conditions. If you are pregnant, you should discuss your immunization record with your obstetrician well before your due date.

Whooping Cough (Pertussis)

CULPRIT The bacterium *Bordetella pertussis* causes whooping cough.

INFECTION INFO Whooping cough is a bacterial infection of the respiratory system marked by severe coughing spells that end in a "whooping" sound when a child takes a breath. These coughing spells can last more than a minute and cause a child to turn purple or red and sometimes vomit. In severe episodes, the child may suffer from lack of oxygen to the brain.

WHO'S AT RISK Whooping cough is highly contagious. It can occur at any age but is most severe before children reach their first birthday, because they are not yet adequately protected by immunizations. The immunity provided by the early childhood vaccines and the booster often wanes, leaving adolescents and adults susceptible. When these older people get whooping cough, they usually have a hacking cough, not whoops.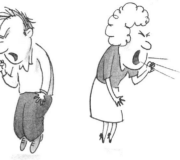

DEFENSIVE MEASURES Whooping cough can be prevented with the pertussis vaccine, which is part of the DTP or DTaP shot. To give additional protection in case immunity fades, the American Academy of Pediatrics now recommends a booster shot of the newer combination vaccine (called Tdap) for those between the ages of 11 and 18 instead of the Td booster routinely given in this age range. The older DTP vaccine contained killed, whole bacteria and commonly caused fever, pain, and redness at the vaccination site. Now, a cell-free vaccine that uses inactivated toxins (toxoids) is used. It is better tolerated, although it does not produce immunity that lasts longer than the older product.

If someone in your family has whooping cough, every member of your household might receive antibiotics. Young children who have not received all five doses of the vaccine may require an immediate booster dose if exposed to an infected family member.

Chapter 4 **Down There** You might not want to talk about them, but infections that occur in the genital area can be just as dangerous and important as others discussed in this book. It's probably been awhile since you last had health class, but you need to shake off your embarrassment to keep your private parts working their best.

Chlamydia

CULPRIT The bacterium *Chlamydia trachomatis*, which can be spread through vaginal, oral, or anal sex, causes chlamydia.

INFECTION INFO Chlamydia affects men and women differently. Women usually experience mild symptoms, including vaginal discharge, painful urination or intercourse, lower abdominal pain, fever, and bleeding between periods. However, untreated chlamydia can cause more serious complications in women, such as pelvic inflammatory disease (PID—an infection of the uterus and fallopian tubes that can lead to infertility) and chronic pain. Symptoms in men include painful urination, penile discharge, a burning or itching sensation at the opening of the penis, and testicular pain, but other side effects are rare. The chlamydia bacteria can cause eye infections in both men and women.

Mothers can pass the bacteria to their infants during childbirth, creating a risk for pneumonia and eye infections in their newborns. Fortunately, a few doses of antibiotics can cure chlamydia. In rare instances, Reiter's syndrome, a disease characterized by arthritis and inflammation of the eyes and urethra, can occur as a reaction to a chlamydia infection. Reiter's syndrome can cause lesions or swelling of the urinary tract and joints.

WHO'S AT RISK Anyone who is sexually active can contract chlamydia, and many people do. The Centers for Disease Control and Prevention (CDC) estimates 2.8 million Americans are infected each year. According to the CDC, certain populations, including those with multiple sex partners and sexually active teenage girls, are more at risk. Young women are more prone to the infection because at a young age, the opening to the uterus, called the cervix, is not fully matured.

DEFENSIVE MEASURES The best way to avoid chlamydia or any sexually transmitted disease is to not have sex. But if you are sexually active, keep relations within the bounds of a long-term, monogamous relationship with an uninfected partner, or at least limit the number of people with whom you have sex. Latex condoms, if used correctly, can reduce the risk of a chlamydia infection.

Sexually active women in their mid-20s or younger should be screened for the disease each year. Testing is also recommended for pregnant women of any age, as well as older women who have multiple sexual partners or a new partner who has not been tested.

Genital Herpes

CULPRIT Genital herpes is primarily an infection of herpes simplex virus type 2 (HSV-2). Herpes simplex virus type 1 (HSV-1) can also cause genital herpes, but this is not as common. (See page 73 for more information about HSV-1.)

INFECTION INFO The virus that causes genital herpes is spread through sexual contact and enters the body through small openings in the skin or mucous membranes. The virus doesn't survive for very long once it's outside the body, so it's highly unlikely you can get infected by touching a toilet seat or other common surface.

The first (primary) episode of genital herpes triggers pain and itching on the skin around the genital area, internally, and sometimes on the buttocks. Soon after, red bumps form and then develop into leaking blisters. Some people with genital herpes have flulike symptoms, including fever. Although the sores typically heal on their own within a month, the virus lurks in the body until it reactivates to cause future (although less severe) outbreaks. Genital herpes may not cause any symptoms, or the signs might be so mild they're unnoticed. The primary outbreak usually occurs about two weeks after the virus is transmitted.

Treatment during primary infection with genital herpes will decrease the recovery time but does not change the possibility of reactivation. HSV-1, if occurring genitally, is much less likely to cause reactivations than is HSV-2.

The virus can be passed to someone else during any type of sex, including oral. Although cases are rare, newborns are at risk for contracting genital herpes during vaginal delivery if the mother has an active infection at the time of the birth. This can cause blindness, meningitis, seizures, brain damage, and even death in the baby. Genital herpes can be treated with antiviral, suppressive medications to shorten and prevent outbreaks. These medications can also reduce, but not eliminate, the risk of transmission during sex. There is no cure for genital herpes.

WHO'S AT RISK Anyone who has sex with an infected person is at risk for contracting genital herpes, but women have a slightly higher risk because the disease is easier to pass from men to women than from women to men.

DEFENSIVE MEASURES Abstaining from sex is the most effective way to prevent genital herpes. If you are sexually active, having a long-term, monogamous partner who is uninfected is best. Using latex condoms can help prevent genital herpes.

All pregnant women should be screened for genital herpes in order to prevent its transmission to babies during childbirth. It is also recommended that women receive an annual Papanicolaou (Pap) smear to check for this and other infections.

Gonorrhea (The Clap)

CULPRIT The *Neisseria gonorrhoeae* bacterium causes gonorrhea.

INFECTION INFO A case of gonorrhea occurs when *N. gonorrhoeae* bacteria are spread to and grow and multiply in warm, wet conditions, such as a woman's reproductive tract and urethra or a man's urethra, as well as the anus, mouth, throat, and eyes. Gonorrhea spreads from person to person during vaginal, anal, or oral sexual contact. Symptoms in women are often mistaken for those of a bladder infection, but can progress to vaginal discharge and vaginal bleeding between periods. Men often have no indications of gonorrhea at all, or they might experience a prominent white or yellow discharge from the penis or pain during urination.

If gonorrhea remains untreated, women can develop PID (see page 60) and become infertile, and men are at risk for epididymitis, a painful testicular condition that also can lead to infertility. Both men and women can experience painful infections in the throat and rectum. The condition can be more serious or even life threatening if the infection spreads to the joints (gonococcal arthritis) or the heart valves (gonococcal endocarditis).

A variety of antibiotics can cure gonorrhea, but there are an increasing number of antibiotic-resistant strains. As with most sexually transmitted infections, newborns can pick up gonorrhea during childbirth and develop eye infections.

WHO'S AT RISK Any person who is sexually active is at risk for gonorrhea. The CDC estimates at least 700,000 people develop new cases of gonorrhea in the United States annually. Teenagers, young adults, and African-Americans contract it the most.

DEFENSIVE MEASURES The best way to prevent gonorrhea is to abstain from sexual intercourse (vaginal, anal, or oral), but the bacterium can also be transmitted when infected discharges or secretions get on hands and then the hands come into contact with mucous membranes. Nevertheless, it is extremely important to cover the penis with a latex condom from the moment sexual foreplay begins.

Remember, you won't be able to tell if someone has gonorrhea just by looking because there might not be any visible symptoms. Testing and open and honest communication are the only ways to know for certain if someone is disease-free.

JEOPARDY IN THE JOHN?

Some people will not, except in emergencies, use a toilet outside their home or an acquaintance's home. Others will sit down on an unfamiliar loo only after covering the seat with toilet paper. And some women will not use a public toilet except by squatting over it without touching the seat.

Should you believe the urban legends? Can you get a venereal disease from sitting on the pot?

It is very unlikely that you will become infected with any disease-causing microbe, such as the organisms that cause herpes, gonorrhea, syphilis, HIV, or hepatitis B and C, from a toilet seat. That's because to contract VD, your "business parts" need to have direct contact with the infecting pathogen, and that isn't likely to happen if you're using the seat the way it was intended.

The "squat" position is not only unnecessary, but it might also be harmful. Squatting can keep the urinary bladder from completely emptying, which can be a factor in developing urinary tract infections.

Human Papillomavirus (Genital HPV, Genital Warts)

CULPRIT The human papillomavirus (HPV) belongs to a family of more than 100 different virus strains, some of which cause warts on toes or fingers. Of these HPV types, about 30 viruses are spread through sexual contact and cause infections in the genital area, including genital warts (condyloma).

INFECTION INFO According to the CDC, about 20 million people in the United States are infected with HPV, and at least half of all sexually active men and women will have an HPV infection at some point in their lives. About 6.2 million Americans get a new genital HPV infection each year. The vast majority of people will never know they are infected because the HPV infection will pass without causing any symptoms. A small group of people will develop genital warts, and an even smaller percentage will see HPV infection lead to precancerous tissue (dysplasia). Although cases are rare, a pregnant woman can pass HPV to her baby during childbirth. The infant then is at risk for developing warts in the voice box or throat.

Everything in the genital area, from the skin of the penis and the anus to the vulva and the cervix, are fair game when it comes to HPV. The warts HPV causes are typically painless and appear as soft, raised, and sometimes cauliflower-shape lumps in the genital area. The discovery of precancerous tissue, however, signals a potentially deadly risk. Either way, the warts or questionable tissue should be removed.

There is a strong link between the dysplasia HPV causes and cervical cancer, making HPV infection of extreme importance for women. However, the strains of HPV that cause genital warts are not the ones that are associated with cancer so the absence of warts is not a "clean bill of health" when it comes to cervical or uterine cancer.

Although there is no cure for HPV, there is a new preventive vaccine. If you already have an HPV infection, a physician or surgeon should treat or remove infected tissue, and then you'll just have to wait for the infection to go away on its own.

WHO'S AT RISK Because they don't always use condoms, teenagers and young adults are most at risk, as are people who have multiple sexual partners. According to the CDC, HPV is the most common sexually transmitted infection in the United States.

DEFENSIVE MEASURES In June 2006, the Food and Drug Administration approved the first vaccine believed to prevent HPV-related cervical cancer, precancerous genital lesions, and genital warts. The vaccine, called Gardasil, is approved for girls and women ages 9 to 26 and is given as three injections during a six-month period. The vaccine only works on certain strains of HPV and is not effective in preventing cervical cancer in women who are already infected by HPV.

Women should talk with their health-care providers about this preventive vaccine but should not abandon other protective measures. One strategy is to either abstain from sexual contact altogether or form a monogamous sexual relationship with someone who is not infected with HPV. Although HPV infection can occur even if a condom is used, the good news is that condom use has been linked with a lower rate of cervical cancer.

You can take other steps to avoid contracting HPV, or at least cut your risk of developing HPV-related complications. These include:

- **Put it out.** If you smoke and become infected with HPV, your chance of developing dysplasia is significantly higher. Plus, nicotine is believed to increase a woman's risk for cervical cancer.

- **Go drug-free.** Using recreational drugs and drinking alcoholic beverages have been known to suppress the immune system; stay away from both to increase your chances of avoiding HPV.

Syphilis (Bad Blood, Lues)

CULPRIT Syphilis is an infection caused by the bacterium *Treponema pallidum.*

INFECTION INFO Although syphilis is curable in its early stages with antibiotics, the disease's oft-silent symptoms mimic a number of other less-troubling diseases and can progress untreated for decades until damage becomes irreversible. Syphilis is spread through direct contact with a syphilis sore—bacteria invade through skin abrasions or mucous membranes in the mouth or genital area. You cannot get syphilis from a toilet seat, towel, doorknob, or any other shared item.

According to the National Institutes of Health, syphilis typically has four stages, and the early symptoms are easy to miss. About two to three weeks after exposure to *T. pallidum*, an ulcer crops up at the very place where the bacterium entered the body. This painless, small, round, and firm ulcer is called a chancre (pronounced "shanker") and appears outside or inside the body. It goes away on its own in about three to six weeks.

About two to three months after exposure, the second phase begins with a nonitchy skin rash on the palms of the hands, the soles of the feet, or other areas of the body. Symptoms mimic a flulike illness and include swollen lymph glands, a sore throat, fatigue, and headaches. Other signs may include weight loss, hair loss, aching joints, and lesions in the mouth or genital area.

The third phase occurs months after exposure. There usually are not visible symptoms during this latent stage, but the infection can be diagnosed with blood tests.

The last syphilis phase can be deadly. At the least, syphilis bacteria cause irreversible damage to the brain, eyes, heart, nervous system, bones, joints, and other parts of the body. The damage can result in mental illness, blindness, deafness, heart disease, brain damage, or spinal cord damage. All of this can occur two to three *decades* after that first small ulcer seemed to disappear on its own.

WHO'S AT RISK Anyone who is sexually active and having unprotected sex is at risk for contracting syphilis, but young adults have a higher syphilis rate. In rare cases, the infection also can be passed from mother to infant through the placenta during pregnancy, causing a disease known as congenital syphilis.

DEFENSIVE MEASURES If you are sexually active, then having mutually monogamous sex with an uninfected partner is the best way to prevent syphilis. Remember, syphilis can be transmitted even when people do not have visible signs of the disease. Keep these tips in mind:

■ **Know your risk.** If you are engaging in risky sexual behaviors, such as having vaginal, oral, or anal sex with multiple partners or having unprotected sex, you should be tested on a regular basis for syphilis and other sexually transmitted infections.

SYPHILIS THROUGHOUT HISTORY

Syphilis was a major scourge in Europe in the late fifteenth and early sixteenth centuries, but there is a great deal of debate about its origins. One school of thought holds that sailors brought syphilis back home from the New World while another says syphilis was always around in the Old World, but it was mistaken for other diseases.

Because it swept through Europe so quickly and with such force, countries blamed each other for its spread:

- The English called the disease the French pox.
- The French called it the Neapolitan or Italian disease.
- The Italians and the Dutch called it the Spanish disease.
- The Portuguese called it the Castilian disease.
- The Russians called it the Polish disease, and vice versa.
- The Turks called it the Christian disease.
- The Persians called it the Turkish disease.
- The Japanese called it either the Portuguese or Chinese disease.

A number of historical figures, including King Charles VIII of France, Ivan the Terrible, writer Guy de Maupassant, philosopher Friedrich Nietzsche, Al Capone, and artist Paul Gauguin, are alleged to have died of syphilis.

- **Beware the bump.** If you have a bothersome bump or a suspicious sore, go straight to your physician. Early diagnosis and treatment is the best way to attack syphilis.
- **Talk about it.** Have open and honest communication with your sexual partner and talk about any history of sexually transmitted diseases.

■ **Keep it covered**. Although latex condoms are not foolproof, they help reduce risk. But according to the CDC, condoms lubricated with spermicides are no more effective than other lubricated condoms in protecting against the transmission of STDs.

■ **Protect your pregnancy.** All pregnant women should be tested for syphilis to prevent congenital syphilis. Syphilis can cause miscarriage, premature birth, stillbirth, or death of newborn babies. Infants who contract congenital syphilis can have deformities, developmental delays, or seizures. The damage caused by syphilis can continue unseen in infants as they grow and lead to the problems of late-stage syphilis, including damage to bones, teeth, eyes, ears, and the brain.

Vaginal Candidiasis (Vaginal Yeast Infections, Vulvovaginal Candidiasis)

CULPRIT Candidiasis is an infection caused by the yeast *Candida albicans*. Although *Candida albicans* is normally present in the body, if an imbalance occurs, the fungus multiplies quickly and causes the symptoms of vaginal candidiasis.

INFECTION INFO A vaginal yeast infection develops inside the vagina and around the vaginal opening when *Candida albicans* begin to multiply quickly. The infection causes intense itching, a thick white discharge, pain and redness, and pain during urination. It's best to seek diagnosis from a physician the first time a suspected infection occurs. Women who have occasional repeat yeast infections usually can get satisfactory treatment from over-the-counter creams and medications.

WHO'S AT RISK The majority of women have at least one bout with vaginal candidiasis during adulthood. Women who are pregnant, have weakened immune systems, or have chronic conditions such as diabetes are at increased risk. Women who use broad-spectrum antibiotics or corticosteroid medications also are at risk because the medications can kill off "good" bacteria and allow *Candida albicans* to thrive.

DEFENSIVE MEASURES There are several measures you can take to prevent a recurrence of vaginal candidiasis:

■ Keep the vaginal area clean and dry. Use unscented soap and don't be tempted to use douches or feminine hygiene sprays. Even something as simple as scented laundry detergent can leave residue on undergarments that irritates the vaginal area and encourage *Candida albicans* to multiply.

■ Avoid tight clothing and opt for cotton underwear rather than nylon underwear. Pantyhose also can trap moisture, which is never a good idea when it comes to preventing yeast infections.

■ Pregnancy changes everything, and your hormones are certainly no exception. Hormonal changes can sometimes trigger yeast infections, so it is especially important to keep the vaginal area dry during pregnancy.

■ Watch your use of medications, especially antibiotics, because they can kill the body's beneficial bacteria and cause a yeast infection. Talk with your physician if you have questions about any medications you take.

■ After swimming or exercising, quickly change out of damp clothing and thoroughly dry the vaginal area.

Chapter 5 Swallowing Scourges

It's hard to put your best face forward when it's covered in sores, or when it feels as though your throat is being attacked by an invader that has a thousand tiny knives. Understanding–and preventing–some of the most common infectious diseases that affect your swallowing will ensure you greet the world with a smile instead of a frown.

Herpes Simplex Type 1 Infections (Cold Sores, Fever Blisters)

CULPRIT Herpes simplex virus type 1 (HSV-1) is to blame, and it causes a contagious infection that can produce cold sores around or, occasionally, in the mouth. (Canker sores, or aphthous ulcers, are different because they only occur inside the mouth. Canker sores are not due to herpes simplex or any identified infection.)

INFECTION INFO Herpes simplex type 1 is transmitted through direct contact between people when they kiss or, for instance, share lip balm or eating utensils. Herpes blisters can form on the lips, gums, roof of the mouth, and throat, then burst and crust over. These sores can linger up to three weeks. Other symptoms include muscle aches, fever, irritability, and swollen neck glands. If a severe sore throat and swallowing problems follow, dehydration might result. This can require a hospital stay, especially for small children.

In many people, after an initial infection the virus can lie dormant in the nerve cells without exhibiting symptoms until it reactivates,

THE TEN PLAGUES OF EGYPT

Is it possible nondivine events could have caused the ten plagues of Egypt, which, according to the Bible's book of Exodus, freed the Israelites from Egypt? Two epidemiologists, John S. Marr and Curtis Malloy, came up with a domino theory in 1996 that was featured in a documentary, *The Ten Plagues of Egypt.* We'll visit their explanations throughout this book.

First plague: ". . . I will strike the water that is in the Nile and it shall be turned to blood. The fish in the river shall die [and] the river itself shall stink . . . ."

During warm weather, certain algae in the water can "bloom." That is, the algae can grow in excessive quantities and produce a red pigment, causing a "red tide" that is toxic to fish and people. Although this usually happens in seawater, the fresh-water in rivers can also be affected. This happened in North Carolina in 1996 thanks to an organism called *Pfiesteria piscidia.*

Second plague: "The [Nile] shall swarm with frogs; they shall come up into your palace, into your bedchamber and your bed, and into the houses of your officials and of your people, and into your ovens and your kneading bowls."

With no fish to feed on their eggs, frogs (probably toads, which can produce thousands of eggs each) could hatch and then exit the toxic river area and enter houses. Away from their normal environment and in great numbers, the toads died.

often because of a stress factor, such as illness with fever, a facial sunburn, the menstrual cycle, or even a toothache. The virus can spread, however, in saliva, even when a person has no symptoms. No medications exist that can eliminate HSV-1, but prescription treatments can shorten outbreaks and help ease pain.

WHO'S AT RISK Anyone can become infected with HSV-1, and almost everyone does, because it is commonly spread among preschool-age children who share food, eating utensils, or drinking glasses.

DEFENSIVE MEASURES There is no cure for HSV-1. In fact, once a person has been infected with the herpes virus, it stays in the body forever. The best medicine, therefore, should be prevention. You can avoid HSV-1 by:

- Avoiding direct contact with sores if someone has an active herpes infection
- Not sharing drinking glasses and eating utensils
- Getting adequate sleep
- Eating a healthful diet
- Avoiding the factors that trigger activation

Infectious Mononucleosis (Mono, The Kissing Disease)

CULPRIT Mononucleosis is a common infection usually caused by the Epstein-Barr virus (EBV), a member of the herpesvirus family. As its nickname implies, kissing can spread the disease, but it can sometimes be transmitted indirectly through mucus and saliva released in the air when an infected person coughs or sneezes.

INFECTION INFO Most people are exposed to EBV during childhood, but the majority will not develop mononucleosis. People who have been infected with EBV will carry it for the rest of their lives, even if they never have recognizable mono. However, EBV can cause serious illness, especially a lymph gland cancer such as Burkitt's lymphoma, in people with compromised immune systems, including those with HIV/AIDS and those on medications to suppress immunity following an organ transplant.

EBV can be found in the saliva for six months or more after a case of mono. Because people carry EBV for life, it can periodically reappear in the saliva. According to the National Institutes of Health, EBV is one of the world's most successful viruses, infecting more than 95 percent of the adult population over time.

A blood test is the best way to diagnose mononucleosis, but common symptoms include fever; sore throat; constant fatigue or weakness; headaches; sore muscles; enlarged spleen and liver; skin rash; abdominal pain; and swollen lymph nodes in the neck, underarms, or groin. Mono is often mistaken for strep throat or the flu.

Mononucleosis will go away on its own in about four weeks, but teenagers and adults might experience fatigue and weakness for several months. If you or your child has an enlarged spleen and swollen lymph nodes, avoid sports for at least a month. An enlarged spleen can rupture, causing abdominal pain and bleeding. Emergency surgery will be necessary if this happens. Antiviral medication is usually not needed to treat mononucleosis, but a physician may prescribe prednisonelike steroids to very sick people with the disease.

WHO'S AT RISK Infants and children younger than 4 who are infected with EBV usually have very mild symptoms or none at all. Teenagers are most at risk for developing mono—the peak ages for infection are 15 to 17.

DEFENSIVE MEASURES There is no vaccine for EBV. However, there are steps you can take to try to prevent mono:

- Wash hands frequently.
- Avoid close contact with those who have mono.
- Do not let your child share cups, bowls, glasses, or utensils with someone who is infected.
- Never allow your child to share a toothbrush.
- Use disposable paper cups and paper towels in the bathroom.
- Do not share toys, teething rings, or similar items.
- Frequently wash and sterilize pacifiers and bottles.
- Disinfect shared surfaces, such as tabletops, kitchen counters, and play equipment.
- Make it clear, especially to teenagers, that kissing a person infected with mono is off-limits.

Strep Throat (Streptococcus)

CULPRIT Strep throat is caused by the bacterium *Streptococcus pyogenes* (group A *Streptococcus*).

INFECTION INFO Although a sore throat is a telltale symptom of strep throat, not all sore throats are caused by this bacterial infection. In fact, most sore throats are the result of viruses. Other strep throat symptoms include red and white patches in the throat; lower stomach pain; fever; general discomfort, uneasiness,

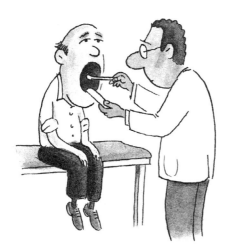

or an ill feeling; loss of appetite; nausea; difficulty swallowing; tender or swollen lymph nodes in the neck; red and enlarged tonsils; headache; and a rash that is often worse under the arms and in skin creases (scarlet fever).

Strep throat responds quickly to antibiotics. Although the illness is relatively common, that doesn't mean it can't be dangerous. Untreated strep throat can lead to the serious disease rheumatic fever (see page 141 for more about this condition), although this happens only in rare cases.

WHO'S AT RISK Anyone can get strep throat, but it is most common in children who are between the ages of 5 and 15. Watch for strep during the school year, particularly during the winter months when large groups of children and teenagers are in close quarters. Your physician will need to diagnose strep throat using a laboratory test, such as a throat culture.

DEFENSIVE MEASURES The most effective way to keep clear of strep throat is to wash your hands thoroughly (or at the very least use a liquid antibacterial hand sanitizer) and push the practice on your kids. The bacterium that causes strep throat hangs out in the nose and throat like 15-year-olds at the mall, so when someone who is infected coughs or sneezes, that gunk can potentially be spread to everything they come in contact with.

If someone in your family gets infected with strep throat, you can take some other precautions (besides washing your hands often) at home to keep everyone else from feeling as though their throats are on fire:

FEVER FALSEHOOD

Myth: If you can't "break," or bring down, a fever, the cause is serious.

Fact: Viruses or bacteria can cause fevers that don't respond to fever medications. There is no relation to the seriousness of the infection.

■ Don't allow the sick person to share drinks, foods, napkins, tissues, or even towels with other family members.

■ Be sure the sick person covers his or her mouth and nose with a tissue when sneezing or coughing and then throws it away to prevent passing infectious fluid.

■ Keep the sick person's eating utensils, dishes, and drinking glasses separate from everyone else's.

■ Thoroughly wash eating utensils, dishes, and drinking glasses after each use; if using the dishwasher, select the "sanitize," "heat dry," and/or similar options.

■ Never share a toothbrush.

■ Don't kiss anyone with strep throat.

Chapter 6 Respiration Roadblocks

Any infection that makes it difficult to breathe is no laughing matter. You may be able to prevent most respiratory infections by taking some simple precautions, but some might require more proactive measures. Follow the tips here and you'll be breathing easier for years to come.

Bronchitis

CULPRIT Viruses, most likely the same ones that cause a cold or the flu, cause 90 percent of bronchitis infections. Bacteria and pollutants (including smoke and chemicals) are also to blame.

INFECTION INFO The bronchial tubes carry air to the lungs. When their lining comes in contact with a virus or irritant, it gets inflamed, prompting special cells to produce mucus. Along with a cough that brings up yellow or green mucus, bronchitis can cause a low fever, fatigue, wheezing, chest congestion and pain, shortness of breath, and a sore throat. For bacterial cases of bronchitis, your doctor will probably prescribe an antibiotic. Chronic (long-term) cases might require steroids to reduce inflammation. Many people show symptoms of bronchitis about three to four days after having a cold or the flu.

With viral cases of acute (short-term) bronchitis, treating the symptoms and being patient are your best bets for recovery.

Most people recover from bronchitis in two or three weeks, but the nagging cough may stick around longer.

WHO'S AT RISK Infants; young children; the elderly; smokers; those with health issues, such as lung or heart disease, cystic fibrosis, and asthma; and those exposed to pollutants on a regular basis are at greatest risk of developing acute bronchitis.

DEFENSIVE MEASURES The best way to avoid bronchitis is to steer clear of colds and the flu (another reason to get a flu vaccination every year). Otherwise, don't smoke and try to limit your exposure to secondhand smoke. Smoke irritates your bronchial tubes and makes you less resistant to bronchitis-causing viruses. Also, stay away from airborne irritants. If the air quality is particularly low, make plans to spend the day inside, and wear a mask if you'll be working around potentially lung-troubling irritants, such as paint, dust, or other chemicals.

Legionnaires' Disease (Legionellosis, Pontiac Fever)

CULPRIT The *Legionella pneumophila* bacterium causes Legionnaires' disease, an "atypical," but serious, form of pneumonia. "Typical" pneumonia caused by pneumococcus (*Streptococcus pneumoniae*) is typical because it responds well to penicillin but not as well to tetracycline, whereas "atypical" pneumonias respond to tetracycline but not at all to penicillin.

INFECTION INFO You can contract Legionnaires' disease by inhaling water droplets that contain the disease-causing bacteria. The bacteria can be spread through showers, hot tubs, whirlpools, cooling towers, hot water tanks, and the air-conditioning systems of large buildings. *L. pneumophila* is not transmitted person to person. The disease was named after a large outbreak at a Philadelphia hotel during an American Legion convention in 1976.

The disease causes fever, chills, cough, muscle aches, headache, fatigue, chest pain, and sometimes nausea, vomiting, and diarrhea. These symptoms appear two to 14 days after exposure to *L. pneumophila*. The disease is best treated with certain antibiotics (not penicillin), and most people recover with no complications; however, in its most serious form, especially in those who already have lung disease, it can be fatal. Pontiac fever is a milder form of Legionnaires' disease that comes with flulike symptoms that appear about three to five days after exposure. It usually clears up on its own.

WHO'S AT RISK People who are most susceptible are the elderly and those who smoke, have lung disease, or have impaired immune systems.

DEFENSIVE MEASURES Protecting yourself can be difficult because Legionnaires' disease is spread through the environment and not from person to person, but there are preventive steps you can take:

■ **Demand diligent disinfecting.** Taking steps to kill the bacteria before it has a chance to contaminate the water is essential. If you use the shower or whirlpool at a gym or other water-sharing facility and see signs the water or faucets are dirty, tell someone. *L. pneumophila* thrives and grows in stagnant water.

■ **Learn a little history.** If you're planning a stay in a hotel or on a cruise ship (another potential hotbed for Legionnaires' disease outbreaks), ask if there have been any recent pneumonialike illnesses reported. Also ask how the air-conditioning system is maintained and how often it is cleaned (the Occupational Safety & Health Administration recommends twice-yearly cleanings of large systems).

■ **Don't smoke.** Smokers are more likely to get lung infections such as Legionnaires' disease.

Sinusitis (Sinus Infection)

CULPRIT Bacteria, viruses (often from a cold), and fungi can all cause a sinus infection.

INFECTION INFO Sinusitis usually stems from a stuffy nose that is due to a cold or allergies. When the nose isn't draining as it should, mucus builds up and clogs the sinuses, providing a breeding ground for bacteria, viruses, and fungi. When your sinuses get infected, they swell and additional mucus builds up, making you miserable. Because symptoms of a cold and sinusitis are so similar, physicians will normally diagnose sinusitis only if your stuffy head lasts more than seven days.

Along with a runny, stuffed-up nose, sinusitis sufferers may also have tenderness in the area of the infected sinus (there are eight sinus pockets located behind the eyes and nose), yellow or green nasal and postnasal drainage, headache, cough, fever, and bad breath. Sinusitis can clear up without medication, but if the cause is bacterial, your physician might prescribe an antibiotic to speed healing.

WHO'S AT RISK Anyone who gets a cold or the flu is at risk for a sinus infection. Smokers, those with asthma and allergies, people with weakened immune systems, and those with mucus-secreting diseases such as cystic fibrosis are more likely to experience sinusitis.

DEFENSIVE MEASURES Protect yourself from colds and the flu and follow these tips to reduce your chances of getting sinusitis:

THE TEN PLAGUES OF EGYPT, *Cont.*

Third plague: ". . . Gnats came on humans and animals alike; all the dust of the earth turned into gnats throughout the whole land of Egypt."

The gnats (or fleas) could have been any insect. In the absence of insect-eating toads, bugs could proliferate, especially around the stagnant water and decaying plant and animal life of the Nile region.

Fourth plague: "I will set swarms of flies on you and your servants and your people, and into your houses. . . . I will set apart the land of Goshen, where my people dwell, so that no swarms of flies shall be there."

A good candidate for this plague would be the stable fly, a fly that both swarms explosively and bites. With the absence of toads and ample insect breeding areas, the stable fly could have gone through a population explosion. Plus, because the stable fly has a small flying range, the Israelites might not have been affected because they lived farther from the Nile.

- **Keep your nose clear.** If you have a stuffy nose, use over-the-counter decongestants or nasal sprays (carefully follow the package directions), drink plenty of fluids, and use a humidifier to help drain your nasal passages.

- **Nix nasal annoyances.** Smoke, dry air, perfumes, and dust can irritate sinuses, opening the door to infection.

- **Avoid allergens.** Allergic reactions can cause sneezing and overproduction of mucus that can clog your nasal passages. Avoid things you know will set off your allergies.

- **Pass on the pool.** Chlorine is a nasal irritant, and diving can push water into the sinuses. If you're prone to sinus infections after swimming, maybe you should stay dry (or try a nose plug).

- **Take care in the air.** Pressure changes during air travel can be hard on your sinuses. Using a decongestant nasal spray when you fly will keep you breathing easier during and after your flight.

Tuberculosis (Consumption, TB)

`CULPRIT` The *Mycobacterium tuberculosis* bacterium is to blame for tuberculosis.

`INFECTION INFO` Only 10 percent of people who are infected with tuberculosis develop active TB—the severe, contagious form of infection that causes symptoms. The other 90 percent who have a TB infection have no symptoms and are not contagious because the body's immune system holds the bacteria in check. In active TB cases, bacteria most often attack the lungs, but can also invade the kidney, brain, spine, or any other organ.

The infection spreads when a healthy person inhales expelled TB bacteria from airborne droplets released by a person with active TB. Symptoms of active TB usually don't begin for two or three months after exposure, if at all, and include a long-lasting (sometimes bloody) cough, chest pain, fatigue, fever, weight loss, and drenching night sweats. Active TB requires taking antibiotics for six to 12 months to completely kill the bacteria.

WHO'S AT RISK Anyone who is in close contact with people who have active TB disease is especially at risk. In addition, people with impaired immune systems (especially those who are HIV-positive); alcoholics and intravenous drug users; health-care workers; those who work in nursing homes, residential care facilities, and prisons; and those who travel internationally are more likely to either develop active TB or to be exposed to it. Tuberculosis is more prevalent in Africa, Asia, and Latin America.

DEFENSIVE MEASURES If you have been in close contact with a person with active TB disease, get a TB skin test or chest X-ray to determine if you are infected. Even if you just have a positive skin test, you may be given preventative treatment to decrease the risk of TB activating later.

If you are around people who have a greater chance of being infected with TB, such as if you work in a health-care or correctional facility, consider wearing a filtration mask that will help prevent you from inhaling TB bacteria. Finally, eat a healthy diet, get plenty of rest, and exercise so your immune system is in top shape.

Chapter 7 Skeletal Snags

Your bones and joints are the framework for your entire body and support your every movement. But when infection ravages the skeleton, getting around can be a painful experience. Fortunately, you can protect yourself from bone-weakening conditions with a little knowledge.

Lyme Disease (Lyme Arthritis)

CULPRIT The bacterium *Borrelia burgdorferi*, which enters the body through a tick bite, causes Lyme disease and its bone-affecting counterpart, Lyme arthritis. Lyme disease takes its name from Old Lyme, Connecticut, where it was first recognized.

INFECTION INFO Lyme disease symptoms are varied and show up all over the body. Skin rash; neurological issues, including paralysis, memory loss, and mood changes; 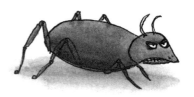 irregular heartbeat; flulike symptoms, such as headache, fever, chills, and muscle aches; and joint pain that can lead to Lyme arthritis are all indications of Lyme disease. The first stage of the infection is a skin rash called erythema migrans, which is a rapidly expanding circular patch, sometimes with central clearing, that occurs within days at the site where the tick was attached.

Several weeks after an infected tick (in the United States, primarily deer ticks and other black-legged ticks) bites a person, the joints swell and then decrease in size, triggering Lyme arthritis, which can later reactivate and again swell the same joints. With time, the joint-swelling episodes become less frequent and don't last as long.

Most cases of Lyme disease can be cured with antibiotics. For some people, however, the joint swelling becomes a long-term condition, although eventually most Lyme arthritis symptoms will go away. In rare cases, people with Lyme arthritis still have symptoms even after long-term antibiotic therapy and may be diagnosed with "antibiotic-treatment-resistant Lyme arthritis."

WHO'S AT RISK Ticks will feed on anyone, so if you're outside in their habitat, you're at risk. The majority of Lyme disease cases occur in the Northeast, northern California, and the Upper

THE TEN PLAGUES OF EGYPT, *Cont.*

Fifth plague: "The hand of the Lord will strike with a deadly pestilence your livestock in the field: the horses, the donkeys, the camels, the herds, and the flocks."

A variety of animal diseases might account for this animal plague. Two, African horse sickness and bluetongue disease, could have been spread by the insects of the third plague and caused the outbreaks. Because the insects transmitting these diseases can't fly far, the Israelites' livestock could have been spared.

Sixth plague: "It shall become fine dust all over the land of Egypt, and shall cause festering boils on humans and animals throughout the whole land of Egypt."

Perhaps the best candidate for this plague is a bacterial infection called glanders. Stable flies (from the fourth plague) can carry glanders, which causes swollen glands and ulcers that may lead to death in a variety of livestock.

Midwest (especially Minnesota and Wisconsin). People who work or otherwise spend a lot of time in wooded areas are more likely to run across the little bacteria-carriers.

DEFENSIVE MEASURES The key to preventing potentially disabling Lyme arthritis is early diagnosis and antibiotic treatment. That said, preventing tick bites or removing ticks from the body promptly will lower your chances of contracting Lyme disease in the first place. Ticks that are removed within 24 hours of when they start feeding rarely, if ever, transmit this infection. For practical tips to prevent tick bites, see the ticks profile on page 177.

Osteomyelitis

CULPRIT *Staphylococcus aureus* is the bacterium that most often causes osteomyelitis. In rare cases, other types of bacteria or fungi also might cause the disease.

INFECTION INFO Osteomyelitis is a fancy word that means bone infection. It typically occurs through direct infection during a traumatic injury (a break or puncture wound) or through bacteria in the bloodstream that travel to and infect the bone. Chronic osteomyelitis occurs when an infection persists due to inadequate treatment or lack of treatment. As a result, the bone doesn't get an adequate supply of blood, and the bone tissue dies. Aggressive treatment requires antibiotics and a surgical procedure to clean up the dead bone.

Osteomyelitis can cause severe pain in the infected area, as well as chills, fever, fatigue, and nausea. Typically, the bones of the legs, upper arms, pelvis, collarbone, and spine are affected.

Antibiotics are prescribed for treatment and are given intravenously at first, and then by mouth.

WHO'S AT RISK People who have diabetes; those who have had a recent trauma, such as a compound fracture (when a broken bone breaks through the skin); people on dialysis; those who use catheters; people who've had orthopedic surgery; and intravenous drug users are more susceptible to osteomyelitis.

DEFENSIVE MEASURES To prevent the kind of osteomyelitis that occurs after injury, practice good hygiene by cleaning any wound or cut with soap and hot water. Hold the injured area under running water for at least five minutes to help flush out bacteria and impurities. Apply an over-the-counter antibiotic cream or ointment to all wounds and cover the site with sterile gauze. Change the bandage often, cleaning the wound each time. If healing doesn't begin quickly, visit a physician.

As for osteomyelitis associated with other diseases, such as diabetes or atherosclerosis, the best prevention is to avoid or properly manage these conditions. Be sure to follow your physician's orders regarding diet, exercise, and medication requirements.

Septic Arthritis
(Bacterial Arthritis, Infectious Arthritis)

CULPRIT Septic arthritis is caused by a variety of bacteria, most often *Staphylococcus* and *Neisseria gonorrhoeae*.

INFECTION INFO Septic arthritis develops either when bacteria spread through the bloodstream from another infected area in

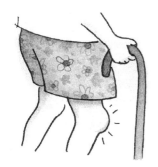

the body and infect a joint, or when the joint is directly infected through traumatic injury or surgery. The condition causes swollen joints (typically in weight-bearing joints such as the knee or hip) and intense pain. Sometimes, the swelling and pain are so severe that they cause partial paralysis. Early diagnosis and treatment with antibiotics is important to stave off long-term damage to the joint.

WHO'S AT RISK People with a chronic illness, an immunosuppressive illness, a bacterial infection, rheumatoid arthritis, a joint injury, an artificial joint implant, and those who've had recent joint surgery are at increased risk. Children, especially those younger than 3, also have a higher risk of septic arthritis.

DEFENSIVE MEASURES Your physician might prescribe preventive antibiotics if you are at high risk for septic arthritis; early treatment is essential to prevent long-lasting joint damage. If you are otherwise healthy and would like to decrease your chances of developing septic arthritis, there are a couple things you can do:

- **Get regular exercise.** A body full of strong, healthy bones, muscles, and joints isn't as prone to developing some kinds of arthritis.
- **Control your weight.** Maintaining a weight that is appropriate for your height and bone structure can help reduce the risk of developing arthritis in load-bearing joints, such as the knees.

Chapter 8 **Liver Liabilities** In old Westerns, when a character accused another of "being yellow," it was an accusation of cowardice. In the real world, however, being yellow might be a sign you've developed a form of hepatitis—a viral infection that attacks the liver, the important organ that aids digestion, filters the blood, and performs a host of other body processes.

Hepatitis A, Hepatitis E (Infectious Hepatitis)

CULPRIT The hepatitis A virus (HAV) and the hepatitis E virus (HEV), respectively, cause these infections.

INFECTION INFO As with other hepatitis viruses, these germs specifically attack the liver, inflaming it and causing it to swell. Both HAV and HEV infections can cause jaundice (yellowing of the eyes and skin; also called icterus), abdominal pain, nausea, fever, and fatigue, but either can occur without jaundice (so-called anicteric hepatitis), as well. Hepatitis A and hepatitis E are short-term infections that go away without treatment, and once you have recovered from them, you can't get them again. The infections often have no symptoms.

HAV and HEV are found in the feces of an infected person and are often spread through inadequately sanitized water supplies. Both viruses can also be transmitted when an infected person skips washing his or her hands after using the restroom and then handles food or eating utensils.

WHO'S AT RISK In the developing world, 100 percent of people have been infected with HAV by the age of 10 because of the lack of adequate sanitation and sewage systems; in the developed world, as much as 50 percent of the population has had hepatitis A by the age of 50. High-risk groups for HAV infection include people who live with an HAV-infected person, people who have had sex with an HAV-infected person, sexually active homosexual men, people with hemophilia or other blood-clotting problems, people with liver disease, drug users, travelers to countries where HAV is prevalent (information is available at the Centers for Disease Control and Prevention's Travelers' Health Web site, www.cdc.gov/travel), and those living in areas of the world with ongoing outbreaks (visit www.cdc.gov/ncidod/diseases/hepatitis/a/index.htm for more information).

Hepatitis E is not prevalent in the United States, but travelers to countries with inadequate water sanitation systems can run into this infection. Pregnant women, especially those in their third trimester, are at greatest risk for experiencing severe complications from HEV infection. In addition, recent information has suggested that HEV can be transmitted to people through contact with animal hosts, such as pigs.

DEFENSIVE MEASURES Being a diligent hand washer gives vital protection against both HAV and HEV. Wash up after you use the bathroom or change a diaper and before you prepare a meal.

Getting vaccinated against HAV is your best defense. The CDC recommends anyone older than 12 months and especially those at high risk of being in contact with HAV get the vaccine. If you come into contact with HAV and have not been vaccinated, you can receive protection from developing the disease through immune globulin, but it must be given within two weeks of contact.

There is no vaccine or immune globulin for hepatitis E, but you can protect yourself by following the tips for eating and drinking while traveling in the travelers' diarrhea profile on page 161.

Hepatitis B and D

CULPRIT The hepatitis B virus (HBV) and hepatitis D (or delta) virus (HDV), respectively, are to blame.

INFECTION INFO These viruses are infectious through contact with blood or certain body fluids, but not through saliva, sweat, tears, or feces. HBV can infect you by itself, but HDV can only infect people who acquire it at the same time as HBV or people who are chronically infected with HBV. Dual infections with HBV and HDV are generally worse than infections with HBV alone.

Many people, especially children, who have acute (short-term) hepatitis B will never show any symptoms. Those who do might experience jaundice, fatigue, headache, fever, appetite loss, nausea, vomiting, abdominal pain (especially on the right side), and dark urine. Most cases of acute hepatitis B go away without specific treatment in a few weeks and don't cause complications.

Some people (about 10 percent of recognized acute cases) go on to have chronic (long-term) hepatitis, which puts them at greater risk for liver damage and diseases such as cirrhosis and liver cancer. Contraction of HDV magnifies hepatitis B symptoms and increases the likelihood of liver damage. Medications to treat chronic hepatitis B can be used in some cases.

WHO'S AT RISK Those at risk include anyone in the health-care, public-safety, or other fields where there may be contact with infected blood; those who have unprotected sexual contact with an HBV-infected person or multiple partners; intravenous drug users; those who might encounter unsanitized needles through body piercing or tattooing; people who are on hemodialysis; and babies born to infected mothers. Those living with an HBV-

THE TEN PLAGUES OF EGYPT, *Cont.*

Seventh plague: "The hail struck down everything that was in the field...both man and beast; and the hail struck down every plant of the field, and shattered every tree of the field. Only in the land of Goshen, was there no hail."

Hail is rare in the Middle East but has been reported, as has snow. Hailstorms can be very localized, and this one seemingly missed Goshen. Much of the Egyptians' harvest was obliterated, and the rest was to soon follow.

Eighth plague: "The locusts came upon all the land of Egypt and settled on the whole country of Egypt, such a dense swarm of locusts as had never been before, nor ever shall be again."

Locust plagues of this magnitude are rare, but they do occur in the area. In fact, one was reported in 1968. John S. Marr and Curtis Malloy theorized that the Egyptians then had to compete with the insects. They had to gather up as much of the crop as they could, even though it was contaminated with dead locusts and their droppings, and store the damp, hail-surviving, locust-contaminated, soiled grain underground, away from the locusts.

infected person and travelers to areas where HBV is common (check the CDC's Travelers' Health Web site for information) also have a higher risk of infection.

DEFENSIVE MEASURES Avoiding HBV will keep HDV away, so kill two birds with one stone by:

- **Getting vaccinated.** The hepatitis B vaccine is more than 95 percent effective and lasts at least 15 years (and perhaps for a lifetime). It is recommended for all newborns and for children younger than 18 years old. Anyone who is at high risk should also get the vaccine. If you're exposed to HBV before you finish the three-shot round of vaccinations, contact your physician; you may be given a dose of hepatitis B immune globulin.
- **Practicing safe sex.** Don't have sex with someone who has HBV, and if you are not in a mutually monogamous sexual relationship, use a condom every time you have sex.
- **Avoiding others' blood.** Don't share needles, whether for IV drug use, a tattoo, or a piercing. You also shouldn't share razors or toothbrushes. Health-care workers need to be very cautious when handling needles or other sharp instruments.

Hepatitis C

CULPRIT Hepatitis C is caused by the hepatitis C virus (HCV).

INFECTION INFO HCV is transmitted primarily through blood-to-blood contact via transfusions or contaminated needles, although it has been spread through sexual contact in rare cases. Transmission to newborn babies from their mothers can occur but is much less common than with HBV. No matter how it is acquired, hepatitis C is the form of viral hepatitis most likely to cause chronic infection. Like HBV, HCV can cause permanent liver damage.

According to the CDC, 55 percent to 85 percent of those infected with HCV will end up with chronic hepatitis C. HCV may linger for decades before an infected person develops symptoms such as jaundice, abdominal pain, appetite loss, nausea, fatigue, and dark-colored urine. But the CDC says 80 percent of people with hepatitis C don't experience any symptoms at all, even though the virus may be slowly invading the liver and possibly causing serious damage. Hepatitis C can be managed with infection-fighting drugs. Many people with chronic hepatitis C die with—not of—the infection.

WHO'S AT RISK Intravenous drug users are at highest risk, as are people who received blood-clotting factors that were made before 1987. Those who received an organ transplant or blood before 1992 (when better testing for HCV was made available) should be tested for hepatitis C. People who've had previous liver problems, babies born to infected mothers, and those who work in jobs where they might be exposed to blood are also at increased risk.

DEFENSIVE MEASURES There is no vaccine for hepatitis C, but if you think you might have been exposed to HCV, being tested can get you on a medication regimen early. Otherwise, avoid blood-to-blood contact, especially by steering clear of unsanitized needles (including those used for tattooing and piercing), others' personal items that might carry blood (including razors and toothbrushes), and intravenous drug use. The CDC estimates that IV drug use accounts for 60 percent of all new cases of hepatitis C and is a major risk factor for infection with HBV.

Chapter 9 **Wound Worries** A battle occurs in your body every time you get a wound. Harmful germs face off against your body's defenders—the white blood cells. When the attacking germs get the upper hand, a mild cut can turn into a more sinister infection. Here are three you need to look out for.

Abscesses

CULPRIT Bacteria usually cause abscesses, but other microorganisms, such as parasites and fungi, can also be to blame.

INFECTION INFO If a harmful invader sets up camp somewhere on your body, the immune system mounts a defense by sending white blood cells, the body's main infection-fighting cells, into the area. The white blood cells surround intruders, keeping them from damaging nearby tissues or organs. As the white blood cells build their protective walls, pus (a collection of fluid, white blood cells, dead tissue, and the enemy organisms) forms. This mass of debris is the abscess.

How you develop an abscess depends on its location. Skin abscesses can form from cuts, punctures, or other skin problems that allow germs to breach the skin. Tooth abscesses typically form when gum disease or a cavity goes untreated. Other abscesses form anywhere enemy invaders collect and white blood cells move to attack.

Skin abscesses are one of the most common types of abscesses. The area around a skin abscess will be hot to the touch, tender, swollen, and red. Tooth abscesses are also fairly common. With one of these, you'll experience pain, swelling of the gums and jaw, and, probably, fever. Other sites of abscesses include the lungs, liver, brain, spinal cord, rectum, and vaginal area (Bartholin's abscess).

Skin abscesses are primarily treated with drainage (lancing); antibiotics play a secondary role (when appropriate). Deeper

THE TEN PLAGUES OF EGYPT, *Cont.*

Ninth plague: "... There was dense darkness in all the land of Egypt for three days. People could not see one another, and for three days they could not move from where they were ...."

The theory is that this was a desert sandstorm, which can cause darkness for days and bury houses. Layers of dust covering the humid, contaminated, underground stores of food would contribute to mold growth on the food.

Tenth plague: "At midnight the Lord struck down all the firstborn in the land of Egypt, from the firstborn of Pharaoh who sat on his throne to the firstborn of the prisoner who was in the dungeon, and all the firstborn of the livestock."

John S. Marr and Curtis Malloy believe the death of the first-born of the Egyptians was related to the toxins produced by molds growing on the food in the storage pits. After the darkness, already starved by the previous plagues, the Egyptians would have gone straight to the stored grain. Those entering and eating first would probably have been the dominant people of the family, including the firstborn. These were the ones likely to be killed by the fungal toxins. Likewise the dominant, firstborn animals would be selectively fed or would have eaten first on their own and also would have succumbed to toxins.

abscesses are treated with antibiotics, but surgical drainage may also be necessary. Severe complications arise when germs from the abscess spread to surrounding tissue.

WHO'S AT RISK Anyone is at risk for an abscess.

DEFENSIVE MEASURES Averting an abscess really depends on where the abscess is located, but in general, healthy living and good hygiene are paramount. To avoid skin abscesses, be sure to properly clean wounds and boils and use an antibacterial or antimicrobial ointment when treating any skin abrasions. To prevent tooth abscesses, brush and floss every day, get regular dental checkups, and avoid cavity-causers, such as sugar-filled foods and drinks.

Cellulitis

CULPRIT Bacteria, most commonly *Staphylococcus* and *Streptococcus*, cause cellulitis.

INFECTION INFO Cellulitis is a bacterial infection of the skin brought on by injury (a cut, burn, or insect bite) or by a skin condition, such as eczema, skin ulcer, or athlete's foot. The infection starts at the outermost layer of skin but may head to underlying tissue and the bloodstream. The infected area (most often on the arms, legs, or face) will swell, turn red, and become tender and painful. Cellulitis is treated with antibiotics, and most people recover with no complications.

WHO'S AT RISK Anyone with an abrasion, wound, or other break in the skin can develop cellulitis, but older people; those with weakened immune systems; and those with conditions that inhibit healing and circulation, such as diabetes and peripheral arterial disease, are at higher risk. People who retain fluid because of edema, those who have surgery that could result in slow lymphatic drainage (the lymph nodes hold the bacteria-fighting white blood cells), people who undergo liposuction or other plastic surgery procedures, and intravenous drug users are also at higher risk.

DEFENSIVE MEASURES Be sure to keep any open wound clean and dry and use an antibacterial or antimicrobial ointment. If you have a condition that puts you at higher risk for cellulitis, be extra diligent about protecting any open wounds and follow your physician's orders for properly caring for your condition. Finally, if you are going to handle fish, meat, poultry, soil, or any other potentially bacteria-laden items and you have an open wound, be sure to wear protective gloves.

Lymphangitis

CULPRIT Bacteria, most commonly *Streptococcus*, are to blame for lymphangitis.

INFECTION INFO Lymphangitis is a bacterial infection of the lymphatic vessels, which work with the lymph nodes to set your body's immune system to work. Potentially harmful bacteria enter your body through a wound and travel to the lymph nodes via the lymph vessels; the lymph nodes then send out the white blood cell cavalry. But when invading bacteria overwhelm the vessels that connect your lymph nodes, or when the lymph

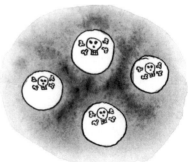

vessels simply aren't able to mount a defense, they become infected, and you get lymphangitis. The condition is typically a complication of cellulitis or a skin abscess and is not the same thing as "blood poisoning," or bacteremia, which is when there are bacteria in the blood.

Symptoms of lymphangitis include chills, fever, rapid heartbeat, and headache, but the telltale signs are red streaks that are warm and tender to the touch and appear underneath the skin in the infected area. The infection can spread to the lymph nodes and cause lymphadenitis. Most people recover completely after a round of antibiotics.

WHO'S AT RISK People who have, or are at higher risk for developing, cellulitis or a skin abscess are at increased risk for lymphangitis. Some dog and cat bites can cause the condition, so those who spend time with furry friends are more susceptible. In addition, some wounds sustained in freshwater environments can lead to lymphangitis, so you have a greater chance of running into this infection if you spend a lot of time at a lake.

DEFENSIVE MEASURES Following the tips for preventing cellulitis and skin abscesses will help protect you from lymphangitis. You also should be thorough when cleaning animal bite wounds, and be sure to use an antibacterial ointment.

Chapter 10 Tummy Troubles

When sitting down to eat, your biggest worry might be getting a touch of heartburn. So you're probably surprised when this simple act leaves you feeling like you've been run over by a truck. If a bout with a foodborne illness has you wondering if you can trust food again, don't despair—you can avoid most culinary creepies with a little awareness and plenty of soap and water.

Botulism

CULPRIT A poisonous nerve toxin produced by the bacterium *Clostridium botulinum* causes botulism. Typically, there are three forms of botulism: You can get it by eating food that is already contaminated with the toxin (foodborne botulism); the bacteria can develop and produce the toxin in the still-developing intestines of babies who ingest botulism spores (infant botulism— mature digestive systems eliminate these spores before they can do any damage); or the bacterial spores can enter the body through a wound, germinate, and produce the toxin (wound botulism).

INFECTION INFO Botulism is a rare, but potentially fatal, infection. Common symptoms include double or blurred vision, drooping eyelids, slurred speech, swallowing problems, dry mouth, and muscle weakness. The toxin causes paralysis that moves from the arms down the body, and it might affect the respiratory muscles, leading to respiratory failure. Babies who develop infant botulism will be lethargic and constipated and have poor muscle tone, a weak cry, and little interest in eating. Foodborne and infant botulism symptoms usually show 18 to 36 hours after exposure to the toxin, but wound botulism symptoms take about a week to appear. Getting treatment for the illness early increases your chance of recovery and can help health authorities pinpoint the cause and keep others from eating contaminated food. Once diagnosed, affected people are treated with botulism antitoxin.

WHO'S AT RISK Botulism is a threat to everyone, but according to the Centers for Disease Control and Prevention (CDC), only about 110 cases are reported each year in the United States. The vast majority of those are infant botulism, which usually affects babies between 6 weeks and 6 months of age.

DEFENSIVE MEASURES Proper food preparation will prevent botulism in most cases. Put these tips to work in your home:

■ **Use caution when canning.** Home canning, especially of foods that have a low acid content, is responsible for most foodborne botulism outbreaks. Be sure to follow proper canning procedures, which you can get from your county extension service. Check with your state's department of agriculture or a university for details.

■ **Refrigerate infused oil.** Oils that are infused with garlic or other herbs can be a ripe spot for botulism toxin production. Keep these products in the refrigerator.

■ **Cool it.** The bacteria that produce botulism toxin thrive at room temperature, so leaving warm food on the counter is an invitation for contamination. The botulism toxin won't begin forming until food is left out for at least 12 hours, but to be safe, don't let your baked potatoes or any other foods sit at

KITCHEN HYGIENE TIPS

- Always wash your hands with hot water and soap before preparing food.
- Wash your hands after handling raw meat, poultry, fish, or egg products.
- Scrub fruits and vegetables with water to remove any left-over pesticides or dirt.
- Remove the outer leaves of leafy greens, such as spinach or lettuce.
- Keep raw meats and their juices away from other foods in the refrigerator and on countertops.
- Use separate cutting boards, utensils, and surfaces for preparing raw meat/poultry, vegetables, and ready-to-eat foods (cooked meat, salad, cold meats).
- Store raw meat/poultry on lower shelves in the refrigerator, beneath other food.
- Keep hot foods hot and cold foods cold.
- Keep pets away from food-preparation areas.

room temperature. Eat them right after cooking or put them in the refrigerator.

- **Keep honey from your little honey.** Honey and corn syrup can be homes for the spores that cause infant botulism. Avoid giving this sweet stuff to babies who are younger than 12 months old.

Clean any wound you have with an antiseptic and watch it closely for signs of infection. Because the botulism toxin only grows in the absence of oxygen, it is very important to keep wounds clean and free of dead tissue. See a health-care provider immediately if you have any concerns.

Dysentery

CULPRIT Dysentery is inflammation of the intestines that causes severe, painful diarrhea. The bacterial form of dysentery, shigellosis, is caused by *Shigella* bacteria (shigellosis is the most common cause of severe diarrhea in the United States). Amebiasis, which is sometimes called amebic dysentery, is much less common and is caused by the one-celled *Entamoeba histolytica* parasite.

INFECTION INFO Both shigellosis and amebiasis are marked by severe, sometimes bloody, diarrhea; fever; and stomach cramps. According to the CDC, about 18,000 cases of shigellosis are reported every year in the United States, but amebiasis usually afflicts people in developing countries. However, cases of amebiasis have occurred in the United States, usually after immigrants from developing countries transmit the parasite, travelers bring it back, or unsanitary living conditions help breed it. Poor hand washing and hygiene habits, especially among children and food handlers, help spread both forms of dysentery. Vegetables harvested in a sewage-tainted field, flies that act as carriers of bacteria, and water supplies and swimming pools can all be sources of *Shigella.*

Unlike most bacterial causes of diarrhea, very few (fewer than 100) bacteria are needed to transmit shigellosis, so it spreads easily from person to person. Besides the infection itself damaging the intestines, *Shigella* bacteria produce toxins that cause further damage.

Shigella bacteria incubate in the body for a couple of days after exposure before symptoms appear, and they generally run their course in five to seven days (although you can still be contagious up to two weeks later). *E. histolytica* can incubate in the body for one to four weeks, and even then, only one in ten infected people will show any sign of illness. If you do get sick, symptoms should resolve themselves on their own, but you should drink plenty of fluids to stay hydrated. You may be prescribed antibiotics for either shigellosis or amebiasis to help lessen the severity and length of the illness.

The long-term outcome of both shigellosis and amebiasis is good. In some cases, shigellosis can cause Reiter's syndrome (see the salmonellosis profile on page 112), and the parasite that causes amebiasis can spread outside the intestines, particularly to the liver.

WHO'S AT RISK Children between the ages of 2 and 4 are the most common victims, as are their families. Anyone who works in a child-care facility or who works or lives in a long-term care facility is also at risk. Children younger than 2 who develop shigellosis may develop a high fever that can cause seizures, but this is rare. Amebiasis cases in the United States are most common to travelers who visit the developing world.

DEFENSIVE MEASURES See our tips in chapter 15 to avoid dysentery while you are traveling abroad. While at home, follow this advice to lower the risk of these diarrhea-causing invaders:

■ **Teach toddlers to lather up.** Educating your little ones about how to wash their hands, and being sure they do so every time they use the restroom, will help you spend less time at the doctor's office.
■ **Ditch the diaper properly.** If your baby has diarrhea, wrap up the soiled diaper in a plastic bag and dispose of it in a garbage

can with a closed lid. After changing the diaper, be sure to wash your hands thoroughly and clean the changing area with a bleach-based household cleaner.

- **Keep the pool clean.** Teach little ones early on that the swimming pool is not a bathroom. When visiting a public pool, know where the restroom is and ask the kids often if they need to use it.
- **Be fickle about your food.** Wash your vegetables and fruits thoroughly before you eat them or cook them.
- **Keep to yourself.** If you have diarrhea, avoid contact with others. In addition, don't cook food or pour water for anyone until your symptoms are gone.
- **Go public.** Letting your coworkers or fellow day-care buddies know about your symptoms may help stop an outbreak. Don't hesitate to let people know about your symptoms as soon as you can so they pay extra attention to their hygiene habits.

Food Poisoning

CULPRIT There are as many as 100 different bacteria that can turn your meal into your stomach's worst nightmare. Some of the most harmful, and most common, foodborne bacteria that cause food poisoning are *Staphylococcus aureus (Staph), Campylobacter jejuni,* and *Clostridium perfringens.* All these bacteria do their damage in your body when you eat food that has been contaminated or handled improperly. *Campylobacter* infection (campylobacteriosis) is a direct bacterial infection that causes diarrhea and is often spread through undercooked chicken. Bacteria-produced toxins cause both *Staph* and *Clostridium* food poisonings. *Staph* toxin most often causes vomiting, and *Clostridium* toxin most often causes diarrhea.

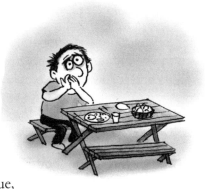

INFECTION INFO Food poisoning symptoms can range from mild to severe, but they typically include vomiting, diarrhea, headache, fatigue, abdominal cramps, and fever. Dehydration is one of the most common complications. The toxin-induced illnesses begin within six to 24 hours of exposure, do not cause much fever, and usually resolve within one to two days. Illnesses related to direct bacterial causes, such as *Campylobacter* and *Salmonella* (see the salmonellosis profile later in this chapter), begin two to four days after exposure, usually cause fever, and might last as long as a week.

WHO'S AT RISK Anyone can get food poisoning, but infants, the elderly, pregnant women, and people with impaired immune systems are especially vulnerable to more severe cases.

DEFENSIVE MEASURES The best rule of thumb is to store your food at the proper temperature and completely cook it because bacteria thrive at temperatures between 40 and 140 degrees Fahrenheit. Habitually washing your hands, surfaces, and utensils when they come in contact with raw food and following safe food-handling guidelines at all times should keep you safe. Keeping picnic foods such as egg salad cold will go a long way toward keeping you out of the bathroom (see the Kitchen Hygiene Tips sidebar on page 105 for more information about food safety).

SAFE KITCHEN TEMPERATURES

Bacteria can grow in temperatures between 40 and 140 degrees Fahrenheit. Keep your refrigerator colder than 40 degrees and follow the table below when cooking meat. Use a food thermometer—inserted at the thickest part and away from any bone—to accurately measure the internal temperature. Avoid rare meats to be safe.

Safe Temperature	Foods
140 F	Reheated cooked foods
145 F	Medium-rare beef, lamb, and veal
160 F	Egg dishes; ground beef, lamb, pork, veal; medium beef, lamb, and veal; pork (including raw ham)
165 F	Ground turkey and chicken, stuffing (cooked alone or in a bird)
170 F	Well-done beef, lamb, and veal; poultry breasts
180 F	Whole chicken or turkey, poultry thighs or wings, and duck or goose

Listeriosis

CULPRIT You can catch this infection from foods tainted with the *Listeria monocytogenes* bacterium, which lives in soil and water. Commonly infected foods include meat; unpasteurized dairy products (especially soft cheeses); and processed foods, such as cold cuts and hot dogs, which can pick up the bacterium after processing. Unlike most bacteria, *Listeria* can actually grow, although slowly, at refrigerator temperatures.

INFECTION INFO Symptoms of listeriosis may not suggest a food-associated cause. Initially, there may be no symptoms or just mild fever and aches. If pregnant women get listeriosis, the disease can cause miscarriage, serious infection in the baby, or even stillbirth. In some cases, the bacteria can spread to the nervous system and cause bacterial meningitis, especially in people whose immune system has been altered by chemotherapy or steroids. Listeriosis can be treated with antibiotics for anywhere from two to six weeks, depending on the health status of the infected person.

WHO'S AT RISK The CDC estimates about 2,500 Americans contract a serious case of listeriosis each year, and 500 people die. Pregnant women are 20 times more likely than healthy adults and children to develop listeriosis. Newborns, the elderly, people with compromised immune systems, and people who are on certain medications (including asthma-treating glucocorticosteroids) all have a higher risk of being severely affected by listeriosis.

DEFENSIVE MEASURES You can prevent listeriosis by practicing safe food-handling and food-preparation procedures (see the Kitchen Hygiene Tips sidebar on page 105 for more information about food safety). If you are pregnant or at a higher risk for the infection, you should give up processed soft cheeses, such as Brie, Camembert, and blue cheese; hot dogs; luncheon or deli meats; smoked seafood, unless it's in a cooked dish; any deli salads, such as ham, chicken, egg, tuna, or seafood salads; and any unpasteurized milk or milk products.

Salmonellosis

CULPRIT Salmonellosis is caused by a number of *Salmonella* bacteria. According to the World Health Organization, more than 2,500 types of *Salmonella* bacteria exist, but the most common are *Salmonella typhimurium* and *Salmonella enteritidis*. *Salmonella* bacteria are transmitted through contaminated food products, such as raw or undercooked poultry, raw eggs, raw or undercooked beef, and unpasteurized milk. They can also be found on unwashed fruit or in food that is prepared on surfaces that were in contact with raw foods and not properly washed. Reptiles are prone to carrying certain *Salmonella* bacteria, so you might get infected if you have a pet snake or turtle.

INFECTION INFO The CDC receives about 40,000 reports of salmonellosis a year, but because most people don't go to the hospital or report their illness, the organization estimates about 1.4 million people are actually infected annually. Salmonellosis affects the intestinal tract and causes nausea, diarrhea, vomiting, fever, abdominal cramps, and headache. Most people with salmonellosis feel better in four to seven days without treatment, although severe diarrhea can require hospitalization for rehydration therapy. In rare cases, *Salmonella* bacteria can travel from the intestines to other organs in the body via the bloodstream, which could lead to death if left untreated. But even in those severe cases, treatment with antibiotics will lead to a complete recovery.

A small number of people with salmonellosis will develop a condition called Reiter's syndrome, a type of reactive arthritis that can cause painful joints, eye irritation, and painful urination. Reiter's syndrome symptoms can last for months or years and can lead to chronic arthritis.

WHO'S AT RISK Anyone can get salmonellosis, but infants, the elderly, and people with weakened immune systems or chronic conditions such as AIDS are most vulnerable to severe cases.

DEFENSIVE MEASURES It is easy to avoid meeting a *Salmonella* bacterium; you just need to follow some commonsense precautions:

■ **Resist raw foods.** You wouldn't munch on a raw chicken leg, but how often do you lick the leftover brownie batter? Caesar dressing, hollandaise sauce, cookie dough, and homemade mayonnaise all contain raw eggs and should be avoided.

■ **Welcome well-done meats.** Although checking your meat to see if it's no longer pink in the middle seems like it should be enough to ensure doneness, it may still be hiding *Salmonella* bacteria. Use a meat thermometer and be sure all meat registers in the safe zone (see the Safe Kitchen Temperatures sidebar on page 110 for more information).

■ **Keep things cool.** Refrigerate eggs, and thaw your meat in the refrigerator and keep it there until you're ready to cook it.

■ **Be a savvy sanitizer.** Wash all surfaces and utensils that come in contact with raw meat or eggs with soap and hot water or a bleach-based household cleaner, and wash your hands immediately after handling raw foods.

FREEZER BURN

Bacteria can survive freezing for long periods, so *E. coli* and friends can cause illness if you don't cook food adequately either before you freeze it or after you defrost it. Some bacteria will even reproduce at low temperatures, including in foods that are defrosted at room temperature. You should always defrost food in the refrigerator or under cold running water.

You can, however, kill higher organisms by freezing at the right temperature. Toxoplasmosis cysts, which cause infections in developing fetuses (toxoplasmosis can be passed through the placenta) or in people with damaged immune systems, can be eradicated by freezing meat for a day in a home freezer set at a high setting. And the infectious forms of trichinosis (a round-worm infection) are killed when pork is frozen at -5 degrees Fahrenheit for 25 days (in a home freezer) or at -22 degrees Fahrenheit for 25 hours (in a commercial freezer).

■ **Leave the lizards (and snakes, turtles, and birds) alone.** Avoid handling reptiles or birds (bird feces harbors *Salmonella*) or any kind of animal feces. If you do have any contact with these animals or with any other animals, thoroughly wash your hands.

■ **Be aware of baby.** Be especially cautious in your food preparation and presentation with babies (and the elderly). Don't cut up the chicken and then feed the little one without taking the time to wash your hands thoroughly in between. Also, never let a baby, or anyone else, drink unpasteurized milk, which can transmit a host of infectious organisms.

Stomach Flu (Gastroenteritis, Viral Gastroenteritis)

CULPRIT The stomach flu is caused by a number of different viruses, but among the most common tummy invaders are the rotavirus and any of a number of strains of noroviruses.

INFECTION INFO "Stomach flu" is a misnomer—influenza, or flu, is an infection of the respiratory system and has nothing to do with the discomfort in your gut that occurs when one of the previously mentioned viruses produce inflammation in your stomach and intestines. The results are usually nausea, diarrhea, vomiting, fever, and abdominal cramps. You also might get a headache, chills, muscle aches, and fatigue.

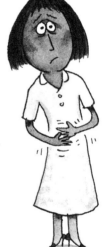

Stomach flu viruses are transmitted through direct contact as well as indirect contact (touching something that's carrying the germs of an infected person, such as a countertop, a toy, or a toilet, and then touching your mouth). Noroviruses can also be spread through food (commonly shellfish, vegetables, and salad greens) and through contaminated water.

Once symptoms begin, the stomach flu usually runs its course in a few days. Because dehydration is the biggest complication of this infection, drinking plenty of fluids is vitally important, especially for children. You should feel much better after a few days and lots of rest, but the viruses can linger in your stool for two to three weeks.

WHO'S AT RISK All stomach flu viruses are highly contagious, but the rotavirus preys almost exclusively on babies and young children. According to the CDC, the rotavirus is the leading cause of diarrhea in infants and young children in the United States and sends 500,000 little ones to the doctor each year. In fact, almost all kids younger than 5 will have at least one bout with the rotavirus. Adults can get the rotavirus, but adult cases are rare and the effects are much milder. Noroviruses attack children and adults.

DEFENSIVE MEASURES These viruses can spread before you even know you're sick, so it's almost impossible to avoid them. You can, however, do your part to keep your home an unwelcome habitat for these digestive dangers:

- **Wash every time.** Because stomach flu viruses abound in stool, it's vital to wash your hands thoroughly every time after you use the restroom or change a diaper. This is especially important if you handle food.
- **To get it clean, use chlorine.** Wash all your surfaces, counter-tops, toilets, sinks, and toys with a disinfectant that has a chlorine base.
- **Be quick to sanitize.** Wash all your soiled clothes, sheets, towels, etc., in soap and hot water immediately after you vomit or have diarrhea.
- **Waste away.** Flush your vomit or stool and keep the area around the toilet clean. If you're caring for an infant or toddler, dispose of diapers quickly and in a sanitary manner.

THE RAW TRUTH BEHIND "OYSTER MONTHS"

An old saying stated that it was only safe to eat raw oysters during months that had R's in their names. This culinary warning suggests that people should keep away from raw oysters during the warmer months of May, June, July, and August.

There were reasons behind the warm-weather ban. In the past, refrigeration was less available and spoilage due to human disease-causing bacteria (both in the water and in the oyster) could more likely occur. In addition, oysters spawn during the summer, and the meat in summer oysters tends to be of lesser quality than the sweeter, plumper oysters of the fall and winter. However, today's farm-raised oysters and better refrigeration technology makes most oysters tasty and disease-free year-round.

Nevertheless, some bacteria in oysters are naturally found in seawater, not just water contaminated by sewage. One bacterium, *Vibrio vulnificus,* lives in the warm seawaters around the U.S. Gulf Coast. Infections caused by this organism are particularly serious and life-threatening in people who have weakened immune systems or liver disease. These individuals should not eat raw oysters at any time of year.

■ **Wash what you eat.** Thoroughly clean your fruits and veggies, and avoid raw oysters and other raw shellfish.

■ **Get out of the kitchen.** Stay away from food preparation until you've been free of symptoms for two to three days.

Tapeworm

CULPRIT The most common tapeworm infestations in people are caused by *Taenia solium* (pork tapeworm), *Taenia saginata* (beef tapeworm), *Hymenolepis nana* (dwarf tapeworm), and *Diphyllobothrium latum* (broad fish tapeworm). The adult forms of these tapeworms live in humans, while the immature forms live in other animals.

INFECTION INFO Tapeworms are acquired by eating uncooked or undercooked food that contains the immature form of the worm. Most people who have tapeworms never show any symptoms. However, when tapeworms cause problems, symptoms might include nausea, diarrhea, stomach pain, loss of appetite, and general weakness. The fish tapeworm can cause vitamin B_{12} deficiency.

People are usually not hosts for the immature (larval) forms of tapeworms, but a complication called cysticercosis occurs when people ingest the eggs of the pork tapeworm, usually through contact with someone who harbors the adult. Cysticercosis can affect the brain and cause seizures. Likewise, echinococcosis (which causes a cyst in the liver and/or lung) occurs when a person ingests the eggs of a tapeworm that generally lives in the intestines of dogs.

Tapeworms are easily treated with medication.

WHO'S AT RISK Tapeworms can infect anyone who eats contaminated food.

DEFENSIVE MEASURES Like most foodborne infections, tapeworms can be avoided through good common sense, such as not eating raw or undercooked beef or pork and practicing good kitchen hygiene. If you're a sushi-eater, the good news is that most fish used in restaurants do not harbor the infectious form of the fish tapeworm.

Trichinosis (Trichinellosis)

CULPRIT Trichinosis is the infestation of the larvae of a parasitical worm species called *Trichinella spiralis.*

INFECTION INFO You can contract trichinosis by eating animal flesh that is infected by *T. spiralis* larvae that aren't killed by cooking. Undercooked pork is a common trichinosis cause, as are game meats, such as bear, fox, and wolf. Trichinosis causes nausea, diarrhea, vomiting, fatigue, fever, and stomach cramps. A headache, cough, swollen eyes, achy joints and muscles, and itchy skin may follow these initial symptoms, and severe cases may cause heart and breathing problems. The first set of symptoms (nausea, abdominal discomfort, and diarrhea) will show up a day or two after eating infected food, but further symptoms (muscle pain and swollen eyes) come around two to eight weeks later. It might take weeks or months to get back to your old self after a bout with trichinosis, but most people do fully recover, either by taking antiparasite medications or by simply allowing the infestation to run its course.

WHO'S AT RISK According to the CDC, only about 12 cases of trichinosis are reported annually in the United States, but anyone who eats raw or undercooked meats, especially game meats, is at risk.

DEFENSIVE MEASURES Be sure you cook all meats until they are safely done (see the Safe Kitchen Temperatures sidebar on page 110 for more information).

THE MANURE GLUT

Animal excrement used as fertilizer is a source of many disease-causing organisms, including *Salmonella, Campylobacter,* and *E. coli* O157. But just how much stinky stuff is out there? In 1997, the Centers for Disease Control and Prevention published estimates of how much manure various types of livestock produce each year in the United States. Cattle were estimated to produce 1,229,190,000 tons, swine 112,652,300 tons, chickens 14,394,000 tons, and turkeys 5,425,000 tons.

The grand total is more than 1.36 billion tons, or 2.72 quadrillion pounds. Even if these numbers were stable (they are likely higher nearly a decade later), this represents approximately 4.5 tons of manure *per person* in the United States.

Chapter 11 Kid Concerns

It's always been tough being a kid, but for those who pick up one of the contagious pestilences often found in preschool or day-care settings, it can be a real pain. But the good news is that few of the viruses, fungi, and microscopic critters that plague youngsters leave the body with serious damage or aftereffects.

Fifth Disease (Erythema Infectiosum, Parvovirus Infection, Slapped-Cheek Disease)

CULPRIT Fifth disease is an infection of parvovirus B19.

INFECTION INFO Despite being called a "disease," fifth disease is actually, in most cases, a mild infection caused by parvovirus B19. This is not the same parvovirus that affects dogs and cats, and it cannot be passed from animals to people or vice versa. The numerical name comes from the fact that fifth disease was among the five rash-associated infections of childhood that were common in the prevaccination era: measles; scarlet fever; rubella; Dukes' disease (also called Filatov-Dukes disease, scarlatinella, and fourth disease), a rash-producing infection not seen today; and fifth disease.

Most people recover from fifth disease quickly without complications. The infection begins with a headache, coldlike symptoms, and a low-grade fever. These symptoms pass within seven to ten days, only to be followed a few days later by the appearance of a bright red rash. However, by the time the rash appears, the infection is no longer contagious.

The rash usually begins on the face, making at least one cheek look like it has been slapped, and spreads in the form of lighter-red blotches to other parts of the body, especially the forearms. Sunlight, heat, exercise, and stress may reactivate the rash until it is completely gone, which typically takes about three weeks. For adults and older teenagers, an attack of fifth disease may create pain or joint swelling in the hands, wrists, knees, or ankles. Parvovirus infection can be worse and more prolonged in adults who have compromised immune systems.

Pregnant women who are not immune to parvovirus B19 should avoid contact with those who are infected because the infection can affect their developing children. Although fifth disease isn't known to cause birth defects, the American Academy of Family Physicians (AAFP) says the risk of fetal death in infected mothers is as high as 10 percent because the virus slows down production of red blood cells.

Remember, by the time the rash develops, fifth disease is no longer infectious. Pregnant women who work in places where parvovirus B19 is more likely to be present, such as elementary schools, should be aware if they are susceptible and consult a physician if an outbreak occurs.

WHO'S AT RISK Any nonimmune person can become infected with fifth disease, but it most often strikes children between the ages of 5 and 15. The distinctive rash is more apparent in children younger than 10.

The AAFP also reports most cases of infection occur in late winter and spring and that it is most easily spread among schoolmates and children in day-care centers. Infection among family members is the second-most common way it gets around.

DEFENSIVE MEASURES There is no vaccine to prevent this infection, but according to the AAFP, studies show that by the age of 15 most people have developed antibodies and are immune, even if they have never shown any detectable symptoms.

> ### CLEAN KIDS
>
> If your children don't wash their hands long enough, teach them to sing their ABCs or "Happy Birthday to You" while doing it. Those songs typically take 15 seconds or more to sing—talk about good clean fun!

Frequent hand washing is a practical and effective method to reduce the spread of this and other viruses. In addition, don't share drinking glasses and utensils, and cover your mouth and nose when coughing and sneezing.

Hand-Foot-and-Mouth Disease (Vesicular Stomatitis with Exanthem)

CULPRIT Hand-foot-and-mouth disease (HFMD) is usually caused by coxsackievirus A16 (named after Coxsackie, New York, where it was first found), a virus that is part of the enterovirus group. Other enteroviruses might lead to HFMD, as well.

INFECTION INFO HFMD is a mild, but highly contagious, infection that starts with a sore throat, low-grade fever, headache, and loss of appetite (infants and toddlers with HFMD can be irritable). The infection is spread through direct contact with the saliva, mucus, blister fluid, or feces of infected people. Within one or two days, sores develop on the tongue, gums, and inside of the cheeks. Likewise, a skin rash of red spots or blisters may appear on the palms of the hands, fingers (especially on the sides), soles of the feet, and, sometimes, buttocks. HFMD is not the same as foot-and-mouth disease (also called hoof-and-mouth disease), which is found in cattle, sheep, pigs, and other animals.

The majority of HFMD cases are minor, and most people recover in seven to ten days without medical treatment. However, dehydration is common because the sores in the mouth can make swallowing difficult. In rare cases, someone infected with HFMD can also develop viral meningitis (inflammation of the membranes and fluid that surround the brain and spinal cord) or other serious diseases, such as encephalitis (inflammation of the brain) and a poliolike illness that causes paralysis. Serious outbreaks of this infection have occurred in Southeast Asia over the past few years.

WHO'S AT RISK HFMD occurs primarily in children younger than 10, including infants, but anyone can contract it. Pregnant women should be especially wary of this disease. Infection at the time of delivery can, in rare cases, cause life-threatening illnesses in a newborn.

DEFENSIVE MEASURES There is no vaccine to prevent HFMD, but standard preventive measures can help. Don't share eating utensils or drinking glasses, avoid close contact with infected people, don't touch blisters or lesions, wash your hands thoroughly and often, cover your nose and mouth when coughing or sneezing, wash and disinfect toys and common surfaces, and keep children who have a fever or open sores away from child-care settings.

Head Lice

CULPRIT The head louse (*Pediculus humanus capitis*) is a tiny wingless parasitic insect that lives among human hairs and feeds on small amounts of blood drawn from the scalp.

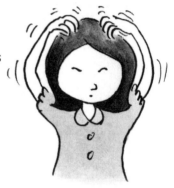

INFECTION INFO Lice lay their eggs (called nits) close to the scalp on individual hair shafts. When the nits hatch, they release nymphs, which resemble adult lice but are smaller. Nymphs are white and look a bit like dandruff, but they can't be removed by brushing the hair. Once the lice are fully grown adults, they become brown or yellow and are more difficult to spot. Lice bites can itch and might cause small red sores that can lead to bacterial infections. Some people who are infected with lice may have swollen lymph glands.

Lice spread easily and quickly among children, especially when kids are in group settings, such as playgrounds, camps, child-care facilities, and slumber parties. Medicated lice shampoos, which kill the insects and their eggs, are recommended for everyone older than 2 years of age with head lice. If you're caring for a child younger than 2, you will need to remove the nits by hand. Some medicated shampoos are not recommended for breast-feeding mothers or for people who weigh less than 110 pounds, so be sure to get your physician's advice before starting a regimen. No matter how you get rid of the insects, it may take a few days for the itching to stop.

WHO'S AT RISK Although anyone can be infected with head lice, children between the ages of 3 and 12 are most at risk. According to findings published in the *Journal of Pediatric Health Care,* girls are more affected than boys because they are more likely to have close head contact and share hair accessories. Because of their hair type, African-Americans are rarely affected by head lice.

DEFENSIVE MEASURES At best, lice don't seem to spread disease; at worst, they are contagious and cause uncomfortable itching. Lice can survive up to 72 hours when away from their food source (your scalp), so you need to kill the ones that haven't made their way into someone's hair. If lice have infested someone in your family, wash all bed linens, towels, and clothing in very hot water and dry them on high heat for at least 20 minutes. Store everything else—pillows, stuffed toys, and similar unwashable items—in airtight bags for two weeks to suffocate and destroy the lice.

After using a medicated shampoo, you can do the following to help prevent a reinfestation:

- For two weeks after treatment, literally go through hair with a fine-tooth comb after shampooing. Lice are immobilized and easier to spot and remove when hair is wet.
- Gather all hair accessories, brushes, and combs and wash them in hot water, soak them in medicated shampoo or rubbing alcohol, or just get rid of them.
- Vacuum all your furniture, carpets, and vehicles. When you are finished, remove the vacuum bag and place it in an airtight container or bag to dispose of it.
- Keep personal care items personal. Remind your children not to share hats, scarves, helmets, combs, brushes, and other items.

■ Avoid bedding, pillows, and carpets if someone who has lice has been on them.

Pinworms (Oxyuriasis, Seatworm, Threadworm)

CULPRIT Pinworms (*Enterobius vermicularis*) are small white worms that live in a host's rectum.

INFECTION INFO Pinworm infections are the most common type of roundworm (parasitic worms) infections in the United States, but they are easily treated. These parasites are easy to acquire—people most often pick them up by unknowingly ingesting pinworm eggs.

According to the Centers for Disease Control and Prevention, pinworm eggs can survive on inanimate surfaces for up to two weeks. The eggs get into the body when someone picks them up from infested surfaces, such as toilets, bath fixtures, countertops, clothing, food, toys, and drinking glasses or utensils, and then touches his or her mouth. After a few weeks, mature female worms move from the intestine to the area around the anus where they lay their eggs.

THE TAPE TEST

If you suspect your child has a pinworm infection, you may need to perform the "tape test" to confirm it. This requires applying transparent adhesive tape to the child's anal region and gently pulling it off. If pinworm eggs are present, they will stick to the tape, which your pediatrician can then examine under a microscope to check for infestation. The tape should be applied and removed first thing in the morning, before showering or a bowel movement, because these actions can remove eggs.

Pinworm-infection symptoms include difficulty sleeping, frequent wiggling or irritability, and an itchy bottom. The persistent itching is caused by the female pinworm when she comes out of the rectum to lay eggs around the child's anus. When the child scratches the itchy area, the minuscule eggs can get under finger-nails and are then easily spread around a home, school, or play area. In rare instances, adults have become infected as they remove or shake bed linens and inhale the eggs.

If you suspect a pinworm infection, look for the little parasites at night, when they lay their eggs. You can sometimes see the worms, which are typically a half-inch long or smaller, around the child's anus or in the bowel movements.

Pinworms can be treated with mebendazole (Vermox), which is packaged in chewable tablets. The tablets are given in two doses two weeks apart. Other medicines, such as pyrantel (Pin-X, Ascarel), are available in liquid or capsule form and are also taken in two doses, two weeks apart.

WHO'S AT RISK People of any age are at risk, but school-age children and preschool-age children are most susceptible to pin-worm infections.

DEFENSIVE MEASURES To prevent the spread of pinworms, everyone in a household where someone is infected should be treated with pinworm medicine. In addition, pinworm prevention should include:

■ Washing hands before a meal and after using the bathroom
■ Washing hands after changing diapers or helping toddlers wipe after bowel movements

- Keeping fingernails short and trimming them often
- Discouraging nail-biting
- Refraining from scratching the anal area
- Changing into clean, freshly washed underwear each day

OTHER INTESTINAL ROUNDWORM INFECTIONS

There are more than 20,000 different kinds of roundworms, most of which are parasitic, living off of people, animals, insects, or plants, depending on the particular species. Two common intestinal human roundworm diseases are ascariasis and hookworm.

Ascariasis is an infection of ascarid worms and is acquired by ingesting eggs excreted in human feces (in areas with poor sanitation, the soil is often contaminated with human feces). The eggs hatch and the small larval forms of the worm migrate to the lungs, where they ascend to the throat and are swallowed. The worms grow into adults in the intestines, and the process starts again. Most ascariasis cases have no symptoms, but a large mass of worms can cause intestinal obstruction. Ascariasis is usually diagnosed by a stool examination or when an earthworm-size adult ascarid is passed in the stool or vomit.

Hookworm eggs that were laid in an infected host travel in feces and hatch into larvae in warm, moist, shaded soil. These tiny larvae penetrate the skin of a new host, often through bare feet. The larvae are carried to the lungs and then move to the intestines, much like ascarids do. The larvae develop into half-inch-long worms in the small intestine, attach to the intestine wall, and suck blood. Most infestations do not manifest symptoms, but large numbers of hookworms can cause anemia.

Both infections can be treated with medication.

If you do get infected, you should use freshly laundered bedclothes and bedding each night; bathe each morning to reduce egg contamination; and open bedroom curtains, blinds, and windows during the day because pinworm eggs are sensitive to sunlight.

Ringworm

CULPRIT Despite its name, ringworm is not an infestation by a worm but a fungal infection of the skin. Different fungi cause ringworm on different parts of the body: *Tinea capitis* (scalp), *Tinea corporis* (body), *Tinea cruris* (groin), *Tinea pedis* (feet), and *Tinea unguium* (nails). These are dermatophytes—fungi that cause infections of the skin, hair, and nails.

INFECTION INFO Ringworm usually appears as red blotches that slowly grow larger, then become itchy and clear in the middle, thus eventually looking like rings. The infection spreads through close contact with infected people or animals; through objects, such as floors, that harbor the fungus; and, rarely, through the soil.

Although testing is not usually necessary, a fungal culture can confirm a ringworm diagnosis. If ringworm is on the scalp, it can cause bald spots. An infection here typically requires oral antifungal medication for an extended period of time, usually six to eight weeks. Ringworm on the nails also requires oral medication, often for several months. Ringworm on other parts of the body is more easily treated—an antifungal cream will clear up the infection in two to four weeks.

WHO'S AT RISK Anyone can develop ringworm, but young children, people who are in close contact with infected individuals or animals, and people with poor hygiene habits are most susceptible.

DEFENSIVE MEASURES Ringworm can be contagious even before symptoms appear, which makes it difficult to avoid. However, you can take a few simple measures to prevent the spread of ringworm, including:

- Treating infected people and pets promptly
- Avoiding contact with infected people and animals
- Not sharing personal items, including hairbrushes, clothing, towels, and shoes
- Keeping common areas clean and disinfected
- Bathing daily
- Washing hands frequently
- Laundering an infected person's clothing and linens in hot water

Roseola (Exanthem Subitum, Roseola Infantum)

CULPRIT Roseola is caused by two similar strains of human herpesvirus (HHV), HHV-6 (the usual cause) and HHV-7, that are spread through secretions from the nose and throat. These are not the same strains of herpesvirus that cause herpes in the mouth or genital areas.

INFECTION INFO Roseola begins with coldlike symptoms, which are followed by as many as seven days of high fever. The fever rises quickly, remains high, and then breaks abruptly. This fast-rising fever triggers convulsions called febrile seizures in 10 percent to 15 percent of children who contract roseola.

As the fever breaks, a pink rash appears on the torso and spreads to other parts of the body, including the neck, face, arms, and legs. Spots caused by roseola turn white when touched and may have a lighter-colored ring around them. Roseola typically does not require professional treatment—the virus must simply run its course. However, you should speak with your child's pediatrician about over-the-counter medications to manage the fever and/or if you are unsure that roseola is the cause.

WHO'S AT RISK Young children, primarily those between the ages of 6 months and 2 years, are most at risk. Adults are rarely affected; it is believed that a childhood case of roseola provides lifelong immunity, although repeat cases have been known to occur.

DEFENSIVE MEASURES Roseola is difficult to prevent because infected people who are not yet exhibiting symptoms often spread the virus; by the time a roseola rash is present, the contagious stage has passed. There is no vaccine to prevent the spread of roseola; however, the basic principles of preventing any viral infection apply, including washing hands thoroughly and often and avoiding exposure to those who are infected.

Chapter 12 Potty Problems

Urinary tract infections (UTIs) are uncomfortable and annoying for anyone, but women are particularly at risk. As if painful urination, fever, chills, and severe abdominal and back pain weren't enough, you make so many trips to the bathroom you might wear a path on the floor. However, there are practical tips you can follow to help keep UTIs out of your life.

Cystitis (Bladder Infection)

CULPRIT A variety of microorganisms can cause UTIs, but *Escherichia coli* (*E. coli*) bacteria are the most common cause of bladder infections. *Staphylococcus saprophyticus* (*S. saprophyticus*) bacteria can cause cystitis, as well, and *Proteus mirabilis* (*P. mirabilis*) bacteria can cause UTIs and produce kidney stones.

INFECTION INFO Bacteria that move from the colon to the bladder via the urethra (the tube that carries urine outside the body) often trigger this common UTI. Symptoms can range from mild to awful and include painful urination; a burning sensation during 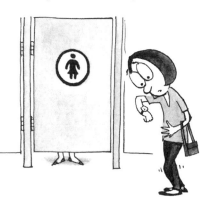 urination; frequent trips to the bathroom (often with very little result); cloudy, blood-tinged, or smelly urine; abdominal pain; and fever. Cystitis may clear up on its own, but antibiotics are often prescribed. If treated, cystitis usually won't result in any complications, but if ignored, the infection can spread to the kidneys (pyelonephritis).

WHO'S AT RISK According to the Centers for Disease Control and Prevention's National Center for Health Statistics, women make more than eight million physician visits a year as a result of UTIs. As many as 20 percent of women have had or will have a UTI in their lifetime, and 80 percent of those women will probably experience a repeat infection in less than a year. Men can get UTIs, too, but they are usually related to obstruction caused by an enlarged prostate gland.

Why are women so unlucky when it comes to UTIs? The female anatomy is one reason. Women have a shorter urethra, which means bacteria have a shorter trip to infect the bladder and other components of the urinary tract. Sexually active women can have bacteria more easily introduced into their urethra, and the hormonal changes pregnant women go through may also contribute to the higher incidence of UTIs. In addition, women who use a diaphragm for birth control also have a higher risk as do those who have a tendency to "hold it" rather than using the bathroom when the urge to urinate hits.

Regardless of sex, anyone who uses a urinary catheter for a prolonged period of time, has experienced changes in their immune system, or has a stone that can block the flow of urine has an increased risk of cystitis and other UTIs.

DEFENSIVE MEASURES Try these simple tips to avoid cystitis and other UTIs:

■ **Get on the juice.** Cranberry juice is a generally accepted way of fighting a bladder infection, but if you don't like the taste, you can try citrus juices. The vitamin C in citrus juices may combat UTIs the same way cranberry juice does.

■ **Drink up.** Drinking lots of water will stimulate urination and help the body flush out bacteria. It also will cause you to make more frequent trips to the bathroom if you tend to wait.

■ **Go when you gotta.** Don't stand around crossing your legs waiting until you're about to burst. Make an effort to use the bathroom as soon as you get the urge.

■ **Practice even safer sex.** Using the bathroom before and after sexual intercourse can help flush out bacteria and drastically lower your chance of getting a UTI. Some physicians will prescribe a single pill of antibiotics to be taken after intercourse and emptying of the bladder to women who have frequent cystitis.

WHICH ANTIBIOTIC IS RIGHT FOR YOU?

When fighting any treatable bacterial infection, the best antibiotic is the one that is most effective against the infecting organism and the one the patient tolerates well. The antibiotic used against one bug may or may not be appropriate for another. Even two people who have the same infection may need to be treated differently because of how their bodies allow penetration of the antibiotic. Other illnesses, existing chronic conditions, and other medications can also affect the appropriateness and choice of antibiotic prescribed.

Your health-care provider will weigh these and other factors when deciding which treatment course to take. Changes may be needed based on lab results and your body's response.

- **Beware of certain birth control.** Using a diaphragm or spermicides that contain nonoxynol-9 might put women at higher risk of developing a bladder infection. If you suffer frequent UTIs, talk with your physician about other forms of birth control.

- **Get in the hygiene habit.** Women should wipe from front to back to avoid transporting bacteria from the colon to the urethra. If you are prone to UTIs, take showers rather than baths and gently wash your vaginal and anal areas with a mild soap. But don't go too far—avoid feminine hygiene sprays and douches.

Pyelonephritis (Kidney Infection)

CULPRIT The same bacteria that cause bladder infections often cause pyelonephritis, but your kidneys can also become infected by bacteria in the bloodstream that travel from an infection in another part of your body.

INFECTION INFO Essentially, pyelonephritis is a UTI, such as cystitis, gone bad. The bacteria that cause the UTI may have been left untreated or were inadequately treated with antibiotics. Those bacteria then make their way up through the ureters (the tubes that connect the kidneys to the bladder) to the kidneys. If you have pyelonephritis, you will have all the symptoms of a bladder infection, but you may also have more intense back and/or abdominal pain, a fever that goes higher than 102 degrees Fahrenheit and lasts for more than a couple of days, chills, vomiting, reddened and moist skin, and fatigue. Elderly people with kidney infections often are mentally confused. Pyelonephritis can be successfully treated with antibiotics.

WHO'S AT RISK Elderly people and people with weakened immune systems are especially susceptible to pyelonephritis, as are those who have recurrent UTIs or a history of urinary tract obstructions, such as kidney stones. Most people who get UTIs will not end up with pyelonephritis if they seek prompt treatment.

DEFENSIVE MEASURES Getting treatment for a UTI as soon as you notice a problem is the best way to avoid pyelonephritis.

TERRIFIC TOILET PAPER

In 1988, the medical journal *Reviews in Infectious Diseases* published an article written by Dr. Walter Hughes entitled "A Tribute to Toilet Paper." It is still one of the few medical publications about the subject that deals with anything besides contact dermatitis from the scented variety. And that's a shame because that thin double sheet of paper acts in concert with hand washing to protect you from millions of potentially harmful bacteria, viruses, and protozoa. Interesting facts from Dr. Hughes's article:

■ Historians think the Chinese were the first to use toilet paper.

■ Seth Wheeler patented the toilet paper roll in 1871.

■ Early toilet paper in the United States was made from the same paper stock as newspapers.

■ Because of shortages during World War II, civilian hoarding of the product was common.

■ The name "toilet paper" was thought to be risqué, and it took until 1975 for the American Broadcasting Company to use that term instead of the more sedate "bathroom tissue."

Chapter 13 Heart Hazards

Serious infections of the heart have nothing to do with being lovesick. Although endocarditis and rheumatic fever are relatively rare, they do require prompt medical attention.

Endocarditis

CULPRIT Bacteria (and sometimes fungi) that enter the bloodstream (a bacterial infection of the blood is called bacteremia) and travel to the heart valves cause endocarditis.

INFECTION INFO Endocarditis is an infection of the endocardium, which is the inner lining of the heart. The infection occurs when microorganisms travel through the bloodstream and get stuck on (usually) an abnormal heart valve, or, rarely, on damaged heart tissue. Once these interlopers begin collecting on the heart valves, they can destroy them.

Symptoms of endocarditis develop about two weeks after infection begins. Endocarditis usually begins with mild symptoms, such as fever and fatigue, that lead to more serious signs, such as weight loss, night sweats, painful joints, shortness of breath, persistent cough, blood in the urine, and petechiae (tiny purple or red spots on the skin). If left untreated, endocarditis can cause heart failure and death. Endocarditis is treated with antibiotics that are usually given intravenously for four to six weeks, but surgery might be necessary if a heart valve is damaged. Some more aggressive forms of endocarditis can destroy heart valves within days if left untreated.

At-risk people need to be aware of situations that can cause bacteremia. Having any kind of dental work or surgery that involves the stomach, intestines, prostate, or gallbladder may increase your chances of developing endocarditis.

WHO'S AT RISK Most people with healthy hearts have a very slight chance of getting endocarditis. However, if you have artificial heart valves, damaged heart valves, congenital heart or valve defects, or if you've had a previous bout of endocarditis, you are more likely to fall prey to this infection.

FINISH YOUR ANTIBIOTIC PRESCRIPTION

Many antibiotic treatment regimens last longer than the amount of time needed to kill the bacteria causing the infection. For instance, most cases of uncomplicated urinary tract infections can be treated for only three days, and many can be cured with only one large dose. Despite this, treatment is often prescribed for seven to ten days. This is done to ensure the infection is completely wiped out—weaker strains of bacteria may be killed quickly, but stronger ones may survive, change, and multiply. Taking the complete prescription will help eliminate all strains in the body. In fact, noncompliance with antibiotic prescriptions is often cited as a reason for the development of drug-resistant "superbugs."

In addition, having leftover antibiotics in the house can be dangerous. The drug may be taken for an infection it is not designed to completely eliminate, which can mask a serious infection or allow bacteria to mutate into a resistant strain. In addition, like food, antibiotics have expiration dates, and taking expired antibiotics can cause side effects. Always follow your physician's instructions when it comes to medications.

ARE YOU REALLY ALLERGIC TO PENICILLIN? PART I

Many people say they are allergic to penicillin in its various forms. When asked how their body reacts, they answer in a variety of ways, many of which don't indicate an allergy at all:

"All I remember is waking up in an ICU with a tube in my throat and hives all over my body."

This is anaphylaxis, a serious and true allergic reaction resulting from hypersensitivity that can lead to shock and respiratory distress. In such individuals, penicillins should be used only when absolutely needed, and then only after a procedure called desensitization, where the allergic person is given gradually increasing dosages of penicillin in a controlled hospital setting.

"I've never had penicillin, but my mother told me to say I'm allergic because my brother is."

No one is born allergic to penicillin; you can only develop an allergy after being exposed to the drug.

"I threw up after taking penicillin for a sore throat."

Gastrointestinal symptoms that occur after taking a medicine are probably not a result of allergies—intolerance is a better description. Some forms of the same or similar drug may be tolerated better.

DEFENSIVE MEASURES Always alert your physician or any other health professional if you are at risk of developing the infection. The American Heart Association has created an endocarditis information wallet card for health professionals that has treatment guidelines. The card is available at www.americanheart.org.

If you are scheduled for dental work or surgery or are getting a piercing or tattoo, talk with your physician. Most of the time, you will need to start on a round of antibiotics before your procedure to keep any enemy bacteria from setting up camp.

Rheumatic Fever

CULPRIT Rheumatic fever is a complication of infection with group A *Streptococcus* bacteria.

INFECTION INFO Rheumatic fever is a rare inflammation of the heart and other body parts (joints, nervous system, and skin) that usually results from a bout with strep throat. People who develop rheumatic fever tend to have an abnormal immune response to some strains of the *Streptococcus* bacterium. As their bodies fight this bacterial infection, inflammation occurs in their joints and the tissues of the heart and its internal valves.

Initial symptoms of rheumatic fever are those of strep throat—sore throat, inflamed tonsils, fever, headache, and aching muscles. Swollen and painful joints (mostly in the knees, elbows, ankles, and wrists) later develop with abdominal pain, skin rash, shortness of breath, and chest pain. Most signs of rheumatic fever appear about one week to six weeks after a case of strep throat.

Complications of rheumatic fever include heart valve damage; heart failure; endocarditis; erratic heartbeats (arrhythmias); and a rare condition called Sydenham's chorea that causes moodiness, weakened muscles, and jerky movements of the face, feet, and hands. Rheumatic fever is treated with antibiotics and anti-inflammatory drugs. People typically recover fully but might need to take low-dose antibiotics for a number of years to prevent any recurrences and further damage to the heart.

WHO'S AT RISK Children between the ages of 6 and 15 (more often girls) are at the highest risk of developing rheumatic fever. Those who have weakened immune systems are also more susceptible.

DEFENSIVE MEASURES Some cases of rheumatic fever can occur following a "silent" strep throat infection that has no symptoms. The best defense against rheumatic fever is to treat a documented strep throat infection with antibiotics as soon as symptoms appear. If sore throat with a fever higher than 101 degrees Fahrenheit lasts more than 24 hours, contact a physician.

Chapter 14 **Thinking Threats** When infections invade the space between our ears, they can wreak havoc with our most important organ—the brain. You don't have to wrack yours for ways to keep your gray matter going strong because we've done the work for you. Read on for helpful ways to keep your noggin healthy.

Bacterial Meningitis

CULPRIT One of three types of bacteria typically causes bacterial meningitis: *Haemophilus influenzae* type b (Hib), *Neisseria meningitidis* (meningococcus), and *Streptococcus pneumoniae* (pneumococcus). A fourth bacterium, *Listeria monocytogenes*, is a less-common cause of meningitis. Finally, newborns can also contract bacterial meningitis, usually from *Escherichia coli* or group B *Streptococcus* in the mother's birth canal.

INFECTION INFO Bacterial meningitis is an infection of the membranes (meninges) and the fluid that surround the brain and the spinal cord (cerebrospinal fluid). Unlike the relatively mild viral meningitis, bacterial meningitis is a serious disease that can lead to brain damage, paralysis, hearing loss, learning disabilities, and even death. The bacteria that cause bacterial meningitis are not highly contagious, but some can be spread through direct, close contact. *Listeria* spreads from contaminated foods and does not pass directly from person to person. Meningococcus infection, with or without meningitis, can cause the spread of bleeding under the skin; this bloodborne infection can be fatal.

Common symptoms include a stiff neck, high fever, headache, nausea, confusion, sleepiness, seizures, and sensitivity to light. These symptoms may be more difficult to detect in infants (and the elderly), but they are often accompanied by poor appetite, listlessness, and fussiness. Treatment for bacterial meningitis requires antibiotics, and the success rate is better when the disease is diagnosed and treated soon after symptoms begin.

Except for *Listeria*, the bugs that cause bacterial meningitis are often present in the throat and mouth on and off throughout a person's life. In people who haven't been immunized against the particular bug and have recently acquired the bacterium, it can penetrate the fluid around the brain and spinal cord. The bacteria then multiply quickly and inflammation sets in, creating the symptoms that mark the infection.

GEOGRAPHY-CHALLENGED INFECTIONS

Some infectious diseases are named for the places where they were first described, but the infection may now occur much more often in other locales. For example:

California encephalitis: This mosquito-spread infection of the brain affects people much more often in the lake areas of Wisconsin. (This variant of California encephalitis is called the LaCrosse virus.)

Rocky Mountain spotted fever: People in the Middle Atlantic states much more commonly contract this bacterial infection spread by ticks.

St. Louis encephalitis: Epidemics of this mosquito-spread infection occur more often in Florida.

WHO'S AT RISK Anyone can contract bacterial meningitis, but it is most common in infants, children, and the elderly. Hib meningitis is most common in children 18 months to 4 years of age, meningococcus meningitis is most common in adolescents and young adults, and pneumococcal meningitis is most common in adults. *Listeria* meningitis generally occurs in people with damaged immune systems, especially those going through chemotherapy for treatment of cancer.

According to the Centers for Disease Control and Prevention (CDC), college freshmen living in dormitories are also at risk for meningococcal meningitis, as are military recruits and those traveling to areas of the world (such as sub-Saharan Africa) where meningococcal disease is more common. Bacterial meningitis is relatively rare in developed countries and usually occurs in isolated cases. Epidemics of meningococcal disease still occur in parts of the developing world.

DEFENSIVE MEASURES Vaccination is the best defense against the three most common causes of bacterial meningitis. Hib bacteria were the leading cause of bacterial meningitis until the 1990s, when Hib-preventing vaccines became a routine part of childhood immunizations (see the invasive H. flu profile on page 47).

Today, with the virtual elimination of Hib meningitis in the developed world thanks to the widespread use of the vaccine, meningococcus and pneumococcus now cause most cases, except for those in newborns. According to the CDC, two vaccines help protect against most, but not all, types of *Neisseria meningitidis,* meningococcal polysaccharide vaccine (MPSV4 or Menomune) and meningococcal conjugate vaccine (MCV4 or MenactraT).

ANTIBIOTIC RESISTANCE

You've probably heard about "superbugs," which are various forms of bacteria that are resistant to antibiotics. Actually, the term should be reserved for organisms with increased disease potential that are able to cause more and faster-developing diseases.

Using antibiotic medicines does not produce resistance. As microorganisms reproduce, genetic mutations randomly occur. Some of these changes cause the organism to die, some have no effect, and others have good or bad effects. The resistant organism becomes prominent because the others that haven't mutated are killed. But remove the drug, and the nonresistant ones may repopulate because the resistant ones may not be as strong if the drug isn't present.

Although antibiotic use may be helpful and even lifesaving, treatment produces some resistance among the normal bacteria that hang out in our skin, mouth, and colon. To minimize resistance, an antibiotic should be used only when necessary, for as long as necessary, and to attack only the infecting organism. Using an antibiotic with a wide spectrum of activity instead of one aimed just at the specific bacterium can be like using an elephant gun to kill a mouse. This problem is prominent in hospitals because antibiotic use is commonplace and "superdrugs" are often used.

MCV4 is recommended for all children at 11 to 12 years of age. For those who have not already received MCV4, a dose is recommended before entering high school. The CDC recommends routine MCV4 vaccination for at-risk people.

The pneumococcal polysaccharide vaccine can be given to ward off meningitis caused by *Streptococcus* (pneumococcus). This vaccine is recommended for people 65 and older or younger people with a variety of chronic diseases or those who've had their spleen removed. A newer vaccine, pneumococcal conjugate vaccine, also is routinely recommended for children. This vaccine may be as active against pneumococcal infection in children as the Hib vaccine was against *Haemophilus influenzae* meningitis.

There is no vaccine to prevent *Listeria* infection. Those susceptible to bacterial meningitis, such as those on chemotherapy for cancer or people receiving treatment to prevent organ rejection after a transplant, should avoid high-risk foods, such as deli meats, hot dogs, and unpasteurized soft cheeses (see the listeriosis profile on page 110 for more information).

Rabies (Hydrophobia)

CULPRIT Rabies is caused by a Lyssavirus, which is excreted in saliva and attacks the nervous system.

INFECTION INFO Without proper treatment, rabies is fatal for almost every person who is infected by it. Most animals have a similar death rate, but some, especially bats, may tolerate infection and survive.

The virus is typically transmitted to people through an infected mammal's bite. The virus travels from the animal's saliva through the person's nerves to the brain, where it can cause inflammation, swelling, and eventually death. The virus descends through nerves and settles in the salivary glands, where it can be passed on through a bite. There have been rare cases of person-to-person transmission via corneal transplants (corneas have many nerves).

Early rabies symptoms, such as headache, fever, and malaise, are not specific to the disease, so contact your physician immediately if you feel these after an animal bites you. As the disease progresses, symptoms can include insomnia, anxiety, confusion, hallucinations, paralysis, excessive salivation, and difficulty swallowing (hydrophobia). If you're bitten by a rabid animal, a series of vaccinations should begin right away. The vaccinations are only effective if given before symptoms develop, which is usually three to four weeks after the bite.

WHO'S AT RISK Those with exposure, accidental or otherwise, to wild animals or free-roaming dogs are most at risk of contracting rabies. According to the World Health Organization, between 30 percent and 60 percent of dog bite victims in areas where canine rabies is endemic are children younger than 15.

DEFENSIVE MEASURES Rabies, although most prevalent in wild animals, such as foxes, skunks, raccoons, monkeys, and bats, can certainly appear in household pets, including dogs, cats, and ferrets. Here are several ways to protect yourself and your family:

■ Rabies may lurk in any "wild" environment, including the woods behind your suburban subdivision. Supervise your dogs, cats, and other pets; keeping them on your property will reduce their risk of exposure.

■ All warm-blooded pets need a rabies vaccination—see your vet and keep these vaccinations current.

■ If you are at high risk for rabies infection, get vaccinated. Veterinarians and wildlife workers routinely receive vaccinations as a precaution.

■ When exploring the great outdoors, keep in mind that overly friendly wild animals are probably just too sick to run away. Enjoy wildlife from a distance and call animal control or a local emergency number if an animal is acting strangely.

■ Do not unintentionally attract animals by leaving the lids off garbage cans, and keep bats at bay by blocking nesting areas on or around your home.

■ Teach your children not to pet or touch animals they do not know, even if the animals seem friendly.

■ If you see a wild animal or a pet foaming at the mouth, stay away and call animal control. When the rabies virus attacks the central nervous system, it makes it difficult for an animal to swallow its own infected saliva, leading to "foaming."

■ If your pet is attacked or bitten by another animal, report the attack to local health or animal control authorities. Even if your pet is vaccinated, your veterinarian will likely recommend a booster shot.

■ When traveling abroad, avoid contact with wild animals and be especially wary around dogs. In developing areas of Asia, Africa, and Latin America, dogs are a major carrier of rabies. Before traveling internationally, talk with your physician about your risk of exposure, whether you should be vaccinated, and what you should do if you are exposed to rabies while in a foreign country.

If you think a rabid animal has bitten you, wash the wound thoroughly with soap and water for at least ten minutes. Note what kind of animal it was and how it was acting. Get medical help immediately and alert animal control authorities to the animal's location.

Viral Meningitis

CULPRIT Viral meningitis is caused by a number of different viruses, many of which are associated with other diseases, such as mumps. According to the CDC, enteroviruses, such as coxsackieviruses and echoviruses, are to blame for most cases of viral meningitis. Mosquitoborne viruses also cause some cases each year.

INFECTION INFO Like bacterial meningitis, viral meningitis is an infection of the meninges and cerebrospinal fluid. Unlike its cousin, however, viral meningitis is usually a relatively mild disease. The viruses that cause it are spread through direct contact with infected people. The CDC estimates there are between 25,000 and 50,000 hospitalizations due to viral meningitis every year.

Sudden symptoms that mimic the flu, particularly in children, are a telltale sign of viral meningitis. These symptoms include fever, headache, vomiting, neck stiffness, and sensitivity to light. Because different viruses can cause the illness, the length of time it takes to heal can vary from just a few days to two weeks.

WHO'S AT RISK Anyone can get viral meningitis, but it occurs most often in children and young adults.

THE URBAN LEGEND OF "RING AROUND THE ROSIE"

Ring around the rosies,
A pocket full of posies,
Ashes, ashes!
We all fall down

This children's nursery rhyme has long been suspected of referring to the outbreak of bubonic plague (the Black Plague) in Europe in the fourteenth century. The usual explanation for the version of the rhyme provided here goes that "rosies" either represent the disease's rash or rosary beads; "posies" were carried to block the odor of plague victims; "ashes" either represent the burning of corpses or the sneezing sounds sick people made; and "all fall down" reflects the profound death rate (25 million people died in Europe, about one-third of the population at the time).

However, the idea that the nursery rhyme refers to the Black Plague is now considered to be an urban legend. According to Snopes.com, a Web site devoted to proving or debunking rumors and legends, the rhyme's history doesn't go back that far—it first appeared in print in 1881. Snopes.com also points to the fact the rhyme has different variations, many of which could never be considered references to the Black Plague.

DEFENSIVE MEASURES Because a virus causes viral meningitis, antibiotics are not an effective treatment. Those who are infected with the virus can be treated at home and usually improve without medical intervention. You can help prevent the spread of viral meningitis by:

■ Washing your hands thoroughly and often
■ Avoiding contact with the saliva or mucus of an infected person
■ Not sharing utensils, cups, and food
■ Disinfecting common surfaces in bathrooms and kitchens with soap and hot water or a bleach-based household cleaner
■ Keeping toys separate and regularly disinfected
■ Avoiding mosquito bites by wearing insect repellent, long pants, and long-sleeved shirts

Chapter 15 On the Road Again

Traveling the world can be hard on the body. Diseases that are a distant memory in the United States may still be commonplace elsewhere. Knowing which microscopic invaders lurk at your destination and making plans to avoid them will help make your trip memorable for the right reasons.

Cholera

CULPRIT The bacterium *Vibrio cholerae* causes cholera.

INFECTION INFO Cholera is a diarrheal illness that can cause severe dehydration; without treatment, cholera can be fatal. You can contract this disease by drinking water or eating food that has been contaminated by *V. cholerae*, often from the feces of an infected person.

If a country has inadequate water and sewage treatment, *V. cholerae* bacteria can spread through rivers and coastal waters. Drinking water or eating seafood from infected sources can spread the infection. Cholera is rarely spread person to person because it takes more than a million bacteria to cause the disease. Outbreaks of cholera occur yearly, especially in Africa during the rainy season.

After they are consumed in infected water and food, whatever cholera bacteria survive the harsh acidic environment of the stomach set up shop in the small intestine, where they reproduce rapidly and create a toxin that causes watery diarrhea. However, not all *V. cholerae* strains produce toxin.

Some people infected by cholera have few or no symptoms, but others react more severely. Diarrhea is the disease's hallmark, but it might be accompanied by vomiting and leg cramps. Only 5 percent of people who get cholera will end up with the most severe symptoms. For those unfortunate few, rehydration is vital, but because the intestines' ability to absorb fluids is not affected, rehydration can be done orally rather than intravenously. Almost everyone who encounters cholera bacteria will recover with no complications.

WHO'S AT RISK Travelers to Africa and Latin America have the greatest risk for contracting cholera. Adequate water and sewage treatment has all but eliminated the disease in the United States, but rare cases occur along the Gulf Coast.

DEFENSIVE MEASURES You can cut your chances of contracting cholera while traveling if you take some precautions:

■ You should wash your hands thoroughly and often to help avoid ingesting and spreading *V. cholerae.*

■ Make good choices when eating and drinking in a foreign country (see the travelers' diarrhea profile in this chapter for more information). The cholera bacterium spreads easily, so being careful about what you eat and drink is your best defense against it.

■ Don't bring any seafood back to the United States.

■ Africa and India have been enduring cholera outbreaks for decades. Before you travel, find out which countries might require you to take more precautions. Get the latest disease information at the Centers for Disease Control and Prevention (CDC) Web site (www.cdc.gov/travel) or call the CDC's Travelers' Health Automated Information Line at (877) 394-8747.

Cutaneous Larva Migrans
(Creeping Eruption, Ground Itch, Sandworm Disease)

CULPRIT Cutaneous larva migrans (CLM) is a human parasitic skin infestation of various types of hookworm larvae.

INFECTION INFO Hookworm eggs found in animal (usually dog or cat) feces hatch and form the larvae that cause CLM. These hookworms are not the same ones that cause human hookworm disease. The larvae live in warm, moist, sandy soil and are determined, sturdy parasites that can penetrate human skin, even through something as seemingly protective as a beach towel.

Much of the time, the larvae enter between the toes, so walking barefoot in soil or sand that is contaminated with animal feces is an avenue for infection. You or your children can also be infected by sitting, playing, gardening, or working in infected soil or sand. The larvae tend to like moist, warm, shaded areas, such as sandboxes and spots underneath houses. You can come into contact with these parasites when traveling to tropical areas in the Caribbean, Central and South America, Africa, and Southeast Asia, but they are also found in the United States in the southeastern and Gulf states.

A few hours after the larvae enter the skin, they form raised red spots on the affected areas (usually the feet, hands, or buttocks). In a few days (or in some cases, a few months), the larvae move under the skin, creating itchy red lines and, occasionally, blisters. These itchy lines usually appear on top of the foot or on the buttocks but can be anywhere on the body that was in contact with the soil or sand. Because the larvae are not from human hookworm, the disease ends at the skin stage. Although it's a very itchy, frustrating infection, most people with CLM will get better without treatment.

WHO'S AT RISK Children are at greater risk of CLM because of their less-than-hygienic play practices. Also at risk are gardeners, sunbathers, utility workers, and travelers to tropical areas.

DEFENSIVE MEASURES The mere thought of CLM probably creeps you out, but you can keep the hookworms from getting a little too close for comfort. When visiting a beach, ask the local authorities if animals are allowed in the area. If no pets are allowed, you have a little less to worry about. And while you're out on the beach, wear shoes or sandals to keep hookworm larvae from penetrating into your feet. You may love the feel of sand between your toes, but you'll hate the feel of CLM even more.

You should also protect the rest of your body while you're on the beach. The parasites that cause CLM can penetrate some objects, so it's a good idea to sit on two or more beach towels, or, better yet, a lounge chair. Finally, stay away from moist, shady, sandy areas because these are the most likely places for parasites to gather.

Dengue (Dengue Fever, Dengue Hemorrhagic Fever)

CULPRIT Any of four dengue virus strains (DEN-1, DEN-2, DEN-3, and DEN-4) transmitted by infected mosquitoes cause dengue (den-GEE). The *Aedes aegypti* mosquito is the most common carrier of dengue viruses.

YOU'RE A HOSPITABLE HOST

Our skin, nose, mouth, and intestines contain variable amounts of what are generally referred to as "commensal" organisms. Generally speaking, these are organisms that, if they stay where they are supposed to be, do no harm. They actually have many useful purposes, including the production of vitamins, such as vitamin K; they keep dangerous bacteria from taking hold; and they stimulate immunity against similar, but disease-producing, organisms. Think of it this way: Commensals eat with you—they don't eat you.

The major hangout for these organisms is the large intestine; in fact, bacteria account for most of the weight of your stool. One study that measured the amount of bacteria per gram of feces (there are 454 grams in a pound) found some interesting results:

■ There are 7.8 million *Escherichia coli* bacteria (the most common cause of urinary tract infections) per gram of feces

■ There are 3,000 *Clostridium perfringens* bacteria (associated with gas gangrene and tetanus) per gram of feces

■ There are 900 million *Bacteroides* bacteria (causes of abdominal abscesses) per gram of feces

INFECTION INFO Dengue is spread when a mosquito bites an infected person and then carries the virus to a noninfected person, passing it on through a bite. After about four to seven days, the person with the virus begins experiencing symptoms that can include headache, backache, fever, nausea, and vomiting. A person with dengue may also develop a rash and complain of joint or eye pain. Younger children tend to have a milder version of the infection than older children and adults.

The viruses that cause the milder dengue infection can produce a more severe form of the disease, called dengue hemorrhagic fever (DHF). People with DHF have a fever that lasts two to seven days and obvious bleeding issues, such as easy bruising, bleeding from the nose or gums, and sometimes internal bleeding. This occurs mostly after second or third infections with dengue strains.

Although there is no treatment for dengue, the illness usually clears up on its own. If any bleeding occurs, be sure to avoid any medications that contain aspirin or ibuprofen to manage dengue-associated fever.

WHO'S AT RISK An estimated 100 million cases of dengue occur around the world every year. Anyone visiting a high-risk country could possibly be exposed to a dengue virus. In general, you're more likely to contract dengue in the South Pacific, Asia, the Caribbean, Central America, South America, and Africa. Dengue-carrying mosquitoes are also more likely to gather in urban areas. But even if you travel to a high-risk area, your chances of being infected with a dengue virus are slight.

DEFENSIVE MEASURES Your best bet to avoid getting dengue is to protect yourself against the mosquitoes that carry the virus. Follow these tips if you're going to be in a high-risk area:

- Cover as much of your body as possible while you're outdoors because the *Aedes* mosquito feeds day and night.
- Use a mosquito repellent that contains DEET and apply it to your body and your clothes.

■ Stay in a hotel that has air conditioning or at least screened doors and windows.

Malaria

CULPRIT Any of four single-celled parasites, *Plasmodium falciparum*, *Plasmodium vivax*, *Plasmodium ovale*, and *Plasmodium malariae*, can cause malaria, a disease of the blood.

INFECTION INFO Female mosquitoes of the genus *Anopheles* spread malaria-causing parasites to people, and the parasites take up residence in your liver. You may show no symptoms of malaria for days, months, or even a year, but the parasite will eventually invade your red blood cells. The cells then rupture, allowing the malaria parasite to invade other red blood cells.

As the red blood cells burst, they release chemicals that cause high fever, chills, headache, muscle aches, and fatigue. Some people might end up with nausea, vomiting, diarrhea, anemia, and jaundice. *P. falciparum* triggers what is considered the most severe manifestation of the disease, which includes seizures, coma, and kidney failure.

> ### FEVER FALSEHOOD
>
> **Myth:** All fevers are bad.
>
> **Fact:** A fever activates the immune system, so it is actually one of the body's protective mechanisms.

If you start having flulike symptoms after visiting a high-risk malaria area, see your physician as soon as possible. Although malaria can be quite dangerous if left untreated, it can be taken care of with prescription drugs. Most people recover fully with treatment and experience no complications.

WHO'S AT RISK Malaria is a serious threat around the globe. According to the World Health Organization, between 350 million and 500 million people acquire malaria every year. The vast majority of these cases happen in the high-risk areas of Central America, South America, Africa, India, the Middle East, Southeast Asia, Hispaniola (the island shared by Haiti and the Dominican Republic), and Oceania (the large region of islands that includes Australia, New Zealand, Indonesia, and Papua New

THERMOMETER HISTORY 101

We tend to take the humble thermometer for granted today, but the invention of this important device has a history that spans hundreds of years. The great inventor Galileo Galilei created a thermoscope in about 1593. This thermometer predecessor used water to indicate temperature differences, but it did not have a scale that measured temperature. Italian physician Santorio Santorio applied a numeric scale to an air thermoscope in about 1612 and is thus credited with inventing the thermometer as a temperature-measurement device.

In 1714, Daniel Gabriel Fahrenheit devised the first mercury thermometer, which was more accurate than the alcohol thermometer that was invented about 60 years earlier. Lord William Thomson Kelvin and Anders Celsius also did their work in the 1700s.

However, it wasn't until about 1867 that British physician Thomas Allbutt invented the modern clinical thermometer. Allbutt's creation improved upon the clunky, foot-long medical thermometer of his time, which often needed 20 minutes to gauge a person's temperature. Allbutt's basic design has been dominant since.

Guinea). Young children, pregnant women, and people with weakened immune systems are most likely to have the worst problems with malaria.

DEFENSIVE MEASURES Some antimalarial drugs kill the malaria parasite while others prevent you from being infected in the first place. If you're traveling to a high-risk area, see your physician four to six weeks before your scheduled departure to get a prescription for antimalarial drugs (and other vaccinations). These drugs work best if you take them on a precise schedule and don't miss any doses.

As with any mosquitoborne disease, your best protection bet is to avoid the critters that carry the infection—in this case, the night-feeding *Anopheles* mosquitoes. Follow the tips in the dengue profile in this chapter to avoid meeting one of these insects.

Travelers' Diarrhea (Montezuma's Revenge, Tourista, Tut's Tummy)

CULPRIT Travelers' diarrhea has a diverse set of causes. Some form of bacteria (most commonly *Enterotoxigenic Escherichia coli*) causes 85 percent of travelers' diarrhea cases; parasites are to blame for about 10 percent of cases; and about 5 percent of infections can be traced back to viruses.

INFECTION INFO Although travelers' diarrhea can be a result of stress due to traveling, jet lag, or change in diet or altitude, the chance is slight. A bacterium, parasite, or virus will almost always be at the root of your traveling tummy troubles. Most people pick up the disease after eating food or drinking water that has been contaminated by feces and not adequately purified. Travelers'

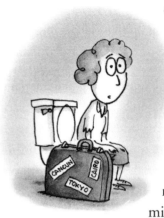

diarrhea usually leads to watery stools, stomach cramps, low-grade fever, and sometimes nausea and vomiting.

Most symptoms will clear up without treatment within a couple of days. If a bacterium causes a case of travelers' diarrhea and the diarrhea persists, antibiotic treatment might be necessary. Travelers' diarrhea rarely leads to any kind of life-threatening condition; the most serious complication is dehydration.

WHO'S AT RISK According to the CDC, ten million travelers end up with a case of travelers' diarrhea each year, and people who visit developing countries in Latin America, Africa, the Middle East, and Asia are most susceptible. For reasons that aren't understood, young adults between 21 and 29 are at a higher-than-normal risk for developing travelers' diarrhea. Children and people with weak immune systems, those with diabetes or inflammatory bowel disease, and people who take acid blockers or antacids (stomach acid destroys bacteria, so without the presence of acid, harmful bacteria can take root) are also more susceptible. Traveling during the summer and during rainy seasons also increases your chance of encountering a nasty bug.

DEFENSIVE MEASURES Although it's not always possible to avoid harmful bugs while you're traveling, these tips should help you keep from getting sick so you can enjoy the sights:

■ **Follow the rules.** The general travelers' rule for eating is: Boil it, cook it, peel it, or forget it. In other words, if you must drink local water, boil it; only eat foods you know have been thoroughly cooked; and stick to fruits with thick skins, such as bananas, that you peel yourself.

■ **Don't drink the water.** This old standard is worth noting because you have to worry about more than just sticking a glass under the tap. Be aware of less-obvious water hazards, such as consuming ice cubes or fruit juices made with tap water, taking a shower, going swimming, or brushing your teeth. Skip anything that may have been washed in contaminated water, such as salads or raw vegetables.

BLEEDING BREAD

One day in the thirteenth century in an Italian church, a sacramental wafer somehow developed spots of bright red "blood." Was this "bleeding bread" a miracle or is there a scientific explanation?

Some strains of the bacterium *Serratia marcescens* can produce a red pigment called prodigiosin. Bartolomeo Bizio, an Italian pharmacist, first described the organism in 1819 as the cause of red discoloration of polenta (a dish made from cornmeal). This discovery was in direct opposition to past claims that bread turning red was a religious miracle related to the blood of Christ.

Bizio gave the bacterium the first part of its name to honor Serafino Serrati, whom he felt had not received proper credit for invention of the steamboat. The second part of its name, marcescens, is Latin for "to decay," and Bizio chose this because of the tendency of the pigment to lose color quickly.

- **Stick to the bottle.** Bottled water, carbonated drinks, beer, or wine in their sealed containers should be okay to drink.
- **Beware the local fare.** Avoid beverages and foods sold by street vendors.
- **Be wary of the unsanitary.** Be sure all food is cooked well and served steaming hot. In addition, don't eat moist foods left at room temperature, and avoid buffets.
- **Think pink.** Bismuth subsalicylate (the main ingredient in Pepto-Bismol) can reduce your risk of developing diarrhea, but there are certain precautions and some strange side effects (like a black-colored tongue). Talk with a health-care professional if you think you might want to take a little pink prevention on your vacation.

Typhoid Fever

CULPRIT The bacterium *Salmonella typhi* causes typhoid fever.

INFECTION INFO Typhoid fever bacteria are usually spread when food or water has been infected with *S. typhi*, most often through contact with the feces of an infected person. Once the typhoid bacteria enter the bloodstream, the body begins to mount a defense that causes a high fever (as high as 104 degrees Fahrenheit), headache, stomach pains, weakness, and decreased appetite. Occasionally, people who have typhoid fever get a rash that looks like flat red spots.

Typhoid fever can be effectively treated with antibiotics. Once treatment begins, improvements start in a few days. Without treatment, the fever can continue for weeks or months, and the infection can lead to death.

WHO'S AT RISK The CDC gets about 400 reports of typhoid fever in the United States each year. However, an estimated 22 million people worldwide get the disease annually. The chances of contracting typhoid fever in the United States are very low; people who travel to developing countries where there is little or no water and sewage treatment or where hand washing is not a common practice are at the highest risk. Prime typhoid fever areas are in India, Asia (especially Tajikistan and Uzbekistan), Africa, the Caribbean, Central America, and South America.

DEFENSIVE MEASURES Because many people who carry typhoid fever appear perfectly healthy and may spread the disease unknowingly, taking extra precautions when you are traveling is essential.

- Wash your hands well and often to prevent the possible spread of bacteria.
- Refer to the travelers' diarrhea profile in this chapter to read the precautions for eating and drinking in developing countries.
- If you are going to be in a country at high risk for typhoid fever or in a rural area where food choices may be limited, typhoid fever vaccines are available. Speak with your physician about getting one and refer to the CDC's Travelers' Health Web site at www.cdc.gov/travel for more information.
- People who have had typhoid fever should not prepare food or drinks for anyone until their stool tests negative for the contagious bacteria.

Yellow Fever

CULPRIT Yellow fever is caused by the yellow fever virus, which is spread by infected *Aedes* mosquitoes.

INFECTION INFO You will begin showing symptoms of yellow fever about three to six days after being bitten by an infected mosquito. These symptoms include fever, chills, backache, nausea, headache, and vomiting. Jaundice, or yellowing of the skin and eyes, is the hallmark of the infection and gives it its name.

Most people recover from yellow fever in three to four days. In more severe cases, the virus might cause bleeding, heart problems, liver or kidney failure, or brain dysfunction. Yellow fever can be fatal. People with the disease may be able to ease their symptoms, but there is no specific medical treatment.

WHO'S AT RISK Yellow fever occurs only in Africa and South America, so only travelers who are destined for these regions need to be concerned about it. The World Health Organization estimates there are 200,000 cases of yellow fever every year (although the organization says the vast majority of cases are not reported), and 30,000 of those cases are fatal. The elderly are at highest risk of developing the most severe symptoms of the infection.

DEFENSIVE MEASURES If you are traveling to high-risk areas of sub-Saharan Africa or tropical South America, you can take some precautions to help keep yellow fever at bay. First, and most importantly, you should get a yellow fever vaccination. Talk with your physician about the vaccine at least two weeks before you travel. The vaccine is only available at authorized locations; call your local health department or visit www2.ncid.cdc.gov/travel/yellowfever to find the one nearest you. Besides getting the vaccine, you should protect yourself from mosquitoes using the tips in the dengue profile on page 156.

Chapter 16 Man's Best Friends

When it comes to companionship, you don't get much better than a pet. Be it feathered or furry, the unconditional love a pet brings to a home can be priceless. But no matter how much you love your pets, you need to know they carry specific germs that can make you and your family sick.

Animal Bite Infections

CULPRIT Any of a number of germs that are found in the mouths of dogs, cats, or wild animals can cause problems for you—particularly such bacteria as *Staphylococcus*, *Streptococcus*, and *Pasteurella multocida*, which can lead to potentially serious wound infections that can spread to tendons, bones, and the bloodstream. As discussed in other chapters, animal bites are also gateways to infection by *Clostridium tetani*, the cause of tetanus (see page 56 for more information) and the virus that causes rabies, an almost-always fatal infection of the brain. (See page 147 for more information.)

INFECTION INFO Your pets may be lovable, but they are animals, so they have the potential to bite. Dogs are much more likely to be aggressive than cats, but cat bites are more likely to cause an infection. Because cats' sharp teeth penetrate farther underneath the skin, as many as 50 percent of cat bites get infected. Wild animals, such as raccoons, squirrels, or rodents, only account for about 5 percent of animal bites each year.

Although animal bites can cause a variety of problems that range from mild skin infections to more serious diseases, such as tetanus and rabies, the vast majority of bites, if treated properly, will leave you with nothing more than a painful reminder to be more careful around animals. If you develop a fever and/or progressive swelling, redness, and pain at the bite site, however, see a physician as soon as possible to be sure you haven't contracted anything through your bite. Likewise, you should visit a physician if you suspect a rabid animal has bitten you.

Follow these steps if you suffer an animal bite:

1. Thoroughly wash the wound with mild soap and water for three to five minutes.
2. Treat the wound with an antibiotic ointment and cover it with a clean dressing.
3. If the bite is on the hands or fingers, see a physician right away. Bites on these body parts are most likely to result in a more serious infection and need to be treated more cautiously.
4. Watch the wound for the next day or two; if there is any redness, swelling, or pain, it may be infected. If so, head to your physician or the emergency room.

WHO'S AT RISK Children have the highest risk of being bitten by animals because they often don't understand the dangers animals can pose. Boys between the ages of 5 and 9 are most likely to end up with an animal bite.

DEFENSIVE MEASURES The most effective way to prevent infection is by curbing risky animal behavior. This requires a two-fold approach: Be sure you and your children know how to deal with

animals, and be sure your pets know how to deal with people.
Follow these tips:

- **Pets need people.** Dogs and cats that are used to being around
  lots of people are less likely to become aggressive when someone new visits your home. Animals that spend too much time
  alone tend to be more belligerent.
- **Don't pet strangers.** You teach your children not to talk to
  strangers, but you also should teach them not to approach or
  pet a strange animal. Even a sweet-looking little kitty can leave
  a nasty bite or scratch.
- **Avoid aggravation.** Teasing his brother is one thing, but teasing the neighbor's dog is another. Be sure kids know not to
  provoke (kick, poke, pull, or chase) an animal. Never bother a
  dog that is eating, sleeping, or otherwise engaged.
- **Send Fido to school.** Send your dog to obedience school to
  learn how to handle aggressive tendencies.
- **Give them a shot.** Be sure your pets are up to date on their
  rabies vaccinations, so even if one of them lashes out, there'll
  be less chance of a serious infection.
- **Neutralize aggression.** Neuter your pets as soon as possible
  (ask your vet about the most appropriate time); pets that are
  neutered are calmer and less likely to react aggressively.
- **Only watch the wild.** Don't go near wild animals. Stay away
  from raccoons, squirrels, rodents, and other outdoor critters,
  even if they are hurt. Animals such as skunks and raccoons are
  nocturnal, so if you see one wandering down the street in the
  middle of the day, chances are good it is sick and you should
  head the other direction and call animal control.

Cat Scratch Disease (Bartonellosis)

CULPRIT The bacterium *Bartonella henselae* causes cat scratch disease.

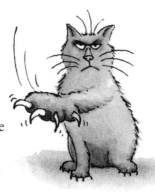

INFECTION INFO You can contract cat scratch disease when a cat infected with *B. henselae* bacteria scratches or bites you. Because the bacteria are found in cat saliva, you can also get the disease if an infected cat licks an open wound on your body. Forty percent of those cuddly cuties carry *B. henselae* bacteria at some point in their lives, but kittens are more likely to harbor them than are adult cats. Felines that spend their entire lives indoors are less likely to transmit the disease.

The first sign that you have cat scratch disease is a bump or blister at the site of the scratch or bite. You might get a mild fever, headache, and just an overall sick and fatigued feeling. After two or three weeks, enlarged lymph glands might develop and can linger for months. Most people will get over cat scratch disease without treatment, but severe cases are treated with antibiotics.

WHO'S AT RISK Anyone who gets scratched or bitten by an infected cat is at risk for cat scratch disease, but those who have a weakened immune system are more likely to suffer serious symptoms, such as appetite loss, weight loss, and an enlarged spleen. These people will likely need to be treated with antibiotics to fully recover.

DEFENSIVE MEASURES Because cats that are infected with the *B. henselae* bacterium exhibit no symptoms, and because the bacterium doesn't make cats sick, it's difficult to know whether yours is infected. However, you can take some preventative measures:

■ Avoid aggressive play with any cat.

■ Some types of fleas carry the *B. henselae* bacterium, so keeping fleas away from your feline can help keep infection at bay. Ask your veterinarian about flea collars or other treatments to keep fleas off your cat. People cannot get the infection from fleas.

■ If you are bitten or scratched, wash the site immediately with mild soap and water.

■ Don't let your cat lick any of your open wounds.

PLANT INFECTIONS–A RISK TO PEOPLE?

Plants are susceptible to infections caused by bacteria, viruses, and fungi just like people are. Can a plant disease organism cause disease in humans? We don't really know, but some organisms can cause infections in both. Whether there is any relationship, and if the same strain of the germ is responsible, is not clear.

One example is a bacterium called *Burkholderia cepacia*, which causes sour skin disease with rot in onions and garlic. The organism has emerged as an important cause of disease in people, especially in those with cystic fibrosis. It is not clear, however, that the strains that affect humans cause onion disease and vice versa.

More may be heard about *B. cepacia* because it is able to degrade a variety of toxic pesticides and herbicides and is able to prevent a variety of plant diseases by suppressing the causative fungus. Could this apparently helpful germ hold a hidden threat to human health? Maybe.

Parrot Fever (Psittacosis)

CULPRIT The bacterium *Chlamydia psittaci* is the cause of parrot fever.

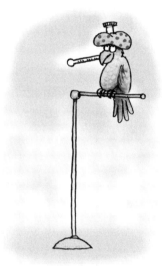

INFECTION INFO Parrots, parakeets, macaws, cockatiels, and lovebirds can all carry the bacterium that spreads parrot fever. More common birds, such as pigeons and doves, can also be carriers. Outbreaks of parrot fever have also occurred in turkey-processing plants. People become infected when they inhale bird remnants, including shed feathers or dust from dried bird droppings, even if the bird itself is not present.

If you've been infected with the parrot fever bug, you will start showing symptoms in about five to 14 days. A moderate case of parrot fever will cause appetite loss and give you a headache, fever, chills, fatigue, and cough. If left untreated, parrot fever can lead to pneumonia (inflammation of the lungs) and affect the liver. Antibiotics will take care of most cases of parrot fever, and the vast majority of infected people recover completely.

WHO'S AT RISK Parrot fever is very rare; in fact, only about 100 to 200 cases are reported each year in the United States. Most at risk are people who handle birds regularly, such as those who have pet birds, pet shop owners, and zookeepers. The elderly and people with weakened immune systems might develop a more severe case of parrot fever.

DEFENSIVE MEASURES If you have a pet bird, keep an eagle eye on your feathery friend. Although some birds infected with *C. psittaci* show no symptoms, some do show signs of illness. Birds with avian psittacosis are lethargic, won't eat, and have ruffled feathers, diarrhea, runny eyes and nose, and green or yellow-green urine. If your bird shows these signs, avoid handling it as much as possible, and visit your vet to get some antibiotics.

You should also clean the birdcage regularly, but be careful when doing so. Wearing a mask and gloves will help protect you from potentially infectious materials. Clean the cage with a disinfectant to kill any harmful bacteria that might be lingering there.

FEVER FALSEHOOD

Myth: Fevers of 104 degrees Fahrenheit to 105 degrees Fahrenheit cause brain damage.

Fact: Even a high fever (which will rarely rise beyond 105 degrees Fahrenheit) will not cause brain damage. Body temperatures need to be much higher (108 degrees Fahrenheit or more) to cause brain damage. However, infections of the brain (encephalitis) or the membranes that cover it (meningitis), can adversely impact the brain no matter what the body temperature is.

Chapter 17 The Little Things

In life, the little things do matter. A parasite that attaches itself to your skin or clothing is certainly one of those little things that will make a big impression on your priority list. Because body lice, scabies, and ticks take time and patience to evict, prevention is the best medicine.

Body Lice

CULPRIT Body lice (*Pediculus humanus humanus*) are parasitic insects that live in clothing and feed on a person's blood. They are different from head lice, which are covered on page 125.

INFECTION INFO Body lice lay their eggs on bedding, on body hair, and in the seams and folds of clothing where body heat enables the eggs to hatch. Because they can't fly or walk, body lice are spread through direct contact with infected people or through contact with bedding, furniture, or other places where the insects have taken up residence. Body lice cause an itchy rash that can turn into bacteria-infected sores.

You can treat body lice infestations by applying a lice-killing shampoo or lotion to your entire body. However, you should check with your physician before using such a product if you are pregnant or breast-feeding. Infected people should bathe in hot water, change into freshly laundered clothes, and wash all infested linens and towels in hot water.

WHO'S AT RISK According to the Centers for Disease Control and Prevention, body lice infestations in the United States are found primarily in homeless, transient people who don't have access to changes of clothes or bathing facilities. Body lice are more common in colder areas where people wear more clothes and in places where war, economic conditions, or other factors may prohibit regular laundering of clothing.

DEFENSIVE MEASURES Body lice can carry diseases such as trench fever and epidemic typhus, but outbreaks are relatively rare. Still, it's a good idea to put up your best defense against these tiny troublemakers:

- Avoid sharing clothes and bedding and keep in mind that body lice can survive for several days on clothing and other items.
- Avoid close, prolonged contact with an infested person.
- Bathe in hot water and use a prescription or nonprescription shampoo or lotion to control lice.
- Wash clothes, linens, and towels in hot water, and either dry them using heat or dry-clean them.

A MITEY BIG PROBLEM

Bird mites parasitize many different domestic and wild birds, including chickens, sparrows, and robins. The bugs normally stay on the birds or in their nests their whole lives, with the adults laying eggs in the nest or on feathers. When birds abandon a nest, the hungry mites freak out and might enter houses in great numbers searching for a blood meal. The mites prefer birds but may confuse you for Big Bird (even if you are not wearing yellow) and chow down. This might make your skin crawl, but it can also make it itch because many mite bites lead to rashes.

Scabies

CULPRIT An infestation of a microscopic mite known as *Sarcoptes scabiei* that burrows in the skin causes scabies. Most cases of scabies are due to the presence of just a few (perhaps ten to 15) mites.

INFECTION INFO Scabies spreads through direct, prolonged skin-to-skin contact or through the sharing of towels, bedding, or clothing. The infestation produces pimplelike bumps or a rash in skin folds near the breasts and on wrists, elbows, knees, shoulder blades, the penis, and the areas between the fingers. A case of scabies can cause intense itching that can be unbearable at night, and scratching can lead to sores that sometimes become infected with bacteria. Prescription lotions will successfully treat scabies, but itching (in part due to an allergy to the mite, alive or dead) might continue for as long as three weeks.

WHO'S AT RISK Scabies affects people of all ages and socioeconomic levels, but it spreads primarily in crowded conditions where people have ongoing skin-to-skin contact. People in child-care facilities, nursing homes, and hospitals, for example, are at increased risk. In addition, the elderly and those with weakened immune systems may contract a severe form of scabies, called Norwegian scabies or crusted scabies, which is an infestation with thousands of mites and is much more easily transmitted to others.

DEFENSIVE MEASURES Preventing scabies is as simple as avoiding close body contact with others who are infested. Another good rule of thumb is to avoid sharing clothing, bed linens, or towels. If in doubt, wash clothes and linens in hot water and dry them on high heat, or press them with a hot iron to kill the mites and their eggs. Wash surfaces such as tables, chairs, and floors, and vacuum all rugs. It's also a good idea to put bedding and stuffed animals in airtight plastic bags for more than 72 hours to starve the little buggers to death. According to findings published in the *New England Journal of Medicine,* mites do not survive more than three days once away from the human body.

Ticks

CULPRIT Ticks are tiny brown mites that, like spiders, are arachnids. Hundreds of different kinds of ticks exist, but dog ticks and deer ticks are very prevalent in the United States.

INFECTION INFO A tick attaches itself to the skin of a human, animal, or reptile and feeds on the host's blood. Each kind of tick usually has a favorite host, and humans are fed on in the absence of a tick's favorite kind of blood. The tick may not be found until after it has enlarged from feeding on your blood, which could take several days.

The immature form of the deer tick is quite small (about the size of a pencil tip) and hard to see, even after it feeds. Despite their small stature, deer ticks transmit diseases, including Lyme disease, that can cause big problems. If left untreated, Lyme disease can spread infection to the heart, joints, and nervous system. The disease has hit every state, but it is particularly common in New England, parts of the Midwest, and northern California. (See the Lyme disease profile on page 87 for more information.)

RODENT WORRIES

Mice, rats, and other rodents aren't just a threat to the food in your pantry; they can spread a number of infections, such as:

Leptospirosis. Leptospirosis is caused by a bacterium that often enters the body through the skin when people are exposed to water contaminated with the urine of infected animals, including rodents, dogs, or livestock. It is not spread person to person. The illness is usually mild, but it can cause serious complications, such as meningitis, pneumonia, liver disease, or kidney disease. Leptospirosis is treated with antibiotics.

Lymphocytic choriomeningitis (LCM). LCM is caused by the lymphocytic choriomeningitis virus, which people usually get from mice (through urine, droppings, and saliva), but infection from hamsters has occurred. Infection can be mild, maybe with just a fever, but viral meningitis, usually not severe, is a possibility. Women who acquire LCM during pregnancy can transmit it to their developing baby, causing complications. There is no specific treatment.

Rat-bite fever. This bacterial infection that is usually associated with a rat bite can cause flulike symptoms, a rash on the palms and on the soles of the feet, and joint pain. Rat-bite fever may also cause a false-positive blood test for syphilis (syphilis has similar symptoms). Most cases resolve within two weeks, but infection can be fatal, especially if it spreads to the heart or brain. It is treated with antibiotics.

Dog ticks are larger and more noticeable than deer ticks; the adults often get as large as one-half inch in length and can enlarge to the size of a marble if left alone. As their name suggests, dog ticks frequently live on the family pet, latching on to ears and other succulent areas. Dog ticks also carry diseases, including Rocky Mountain spotted fever, a bacterial infection characterized by fever, rash, and nausea. If left untreated, Rocky Mountain spotted fever can be fatal.

WHO'S AT RISK Ticks can hitch an unwelcome ride on anyone, but people who spend time outdoors in tall grasses or wooded areas are at greater risk. Being in prolonged, close contact with pets that may be infested with ticks also makes you vulnerable. Always check children for ticks after they spend time in high-risk outdoor areas.

DEFENSIVE MEASURES There's no need to board up the windows and doors and shut yourself in—you can still enjoy the great outdoors despite its smallest inhabitants. You just need to take a few precautions to ensure you don't become a host for these petite parasites:

- Check your pets for ticks if they spend time outside. You should also add a flea and tick collar or other pest deterrent to your pet's hygiene regimen. Your veterinarian can suggest safe and effective products.
- If you are going to walk or hike, stay on a trail rather than venturing through tall grasses, trees with low branches, or piles of dry leaves. Also, stay in areas that get plenty of sun and don't sit directly on the ground.

- Wear long sleeves and light-colored long pants when outside. The extra coverage deters ticks from crawling onto skin, and lighter colors help you see the little bloodsuckers.

- Consider tucking your pant legs into your socks so ticks can't crawl inside. If you are in an area you suspect may be infested with ticks, wear a hat.

- Some experts suggest using a bug spray that contains 10 percent DEET before going into high-risk outdoor areas. Just be sure to wash off the bug spray when you go inside. Although DEET is very effective against mosquitoes, it doesn't have the same success rate when it comes to ticks.

- When you return from walking or hiking, check your clothing and skin for ticks. Run your fingers over your skin and through your hair, and be sure to check your ears, underarms, and groin.

If a tick is latched on to your skin, grab some tweezers and a small vial, such as a film container or small glass bottle. Using the tweezers, grasp the tick as close to its imbedded head as possible, then slowly pull it straight out of the skin. Put the tick in the vial so your physician can identify the species. Some authorities might recommend preventative antibiotics based on the geographic area where the tick was acquired and the kind of tick identified. If done correctly, the tick will usually still be alive after you pull it out of the skin, so be sure the container is closed properly. Wash your hands and watch the bite area for unusual redness or swelling.

Chapter 18 Diabetic Foot Infections

If you have diabetes, you probably work hard to monitor your medications, diet, and exercise, but you might take the health of your feet for granted. Minor discomforts such as corns, calluses, and blisters can lead to serious infections. But don't worry, a few minutes each day, some lotion, and good blood sugar control can help keep you on the dance floor.

Diabetic Foot Infections

CULPRIT Any infection-causing bacteria can cause serious foot problems in people with diabetes.

INFECTION INFO Diabetes is a disease where the body doesn't produce or properly use insulin, a hormone needed to convert sugars into energy. This leads to an excess amount of sugar, or glucose, in the blood, which causes a host of health problems, including foot infections. These infections can be severe enough to require amputation.

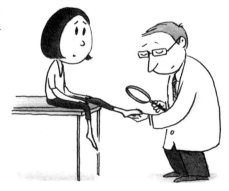

People with diabetes have trouble with their feet for two reasons. First, having excess amounts of glucose in the blood causes nerve damage (neuropathy), and this damage is particularly bad in the feet, where the nerves are the longest. Nerves are the body's alarm system, helping you feel the pain of cuts, blisters, sores, ingrown toenails, and other injuries. But if the nerves in the foot are damaged, the body won't alert you to any problems, and even a severe injury can go unnoticed for days.

Second, people with diabetes are prone to having diseases that affect the large and small arteries, and these diseases can lead to poor blood circulation. Slow circulation means infection-fighting cells and antibiotics take longer to get to the injured area, which lessens their effectiveness. This causes very slow healing and allows bad bacteria to settle into the wound, which turns a minor injury into a major problem.

People who have diabetes get foot infections by not taking proper care of their feet. Those with the disease often have dry, flaky skin that is ripe for cracking. In addition, wearing ill-fitting shoes that cause blisters, neglecting to trim and file toenails, and going barefoot can also lead to any number of minor injuries that can become infected. These infections are worse in people with diabetes because high levels of glucose in the blood feed the infection-causing bacteria and make the problem worse.

If left unnoticed and uncared for, even a minor problem can turn into a serious infection that can spread to the muscle or bone. And if ignored, that infection can get bad enough to cause gangrene (tissue death) and necessitate amputation. Minor foot infections can be treated with antibiotics.

WHO'S AT RISK According to the American Diabetes Association, 20.8 million Americans have diabetes, and every one of them is at risk for a foot infection, especially the elderly. People with

NO-FUN FUNGI

Many different fungi (yeasts and molds) can cause allergic or toxic illnesses or infection. The three fungi detailed here are common infections in the United States, but all are treatable, especially early on. However, the infection will be worse in those with weakened immune systems, including people with AIDS and those undergoing chemotherapy.

Coccidioidomycosis. Coccidioidomycosis is an infection caused by *Coccidioides immitis*, a mold that exists in the soil in the dry or semidry areas of central California and the southwestern United States. Many people are infected by inhaling *C. immitis* spores, but few are affected. The illness usually starts as a self-limited pneumonia, but it can spread to lymph glands, joints, soft tissue, bones, or the meninges (the membranes that cover the brain and spinal cord).

Cryptococcosis. People get this infection by inhaling spores of the yeast *Cryptococcus neoformans*, which is often found in pigeon droppings. Many people won't show signs of the infection, but it can spread to the meninges.

Histoplasmosis. Histoplasmosis is caused by inhaled spores of *Histoplasma capsulatum*, a common species of mold in the upper Mississippi and Ohio River valleys that is often linked to bat caves or abandoned chicken coops. As with coccidioidomycosis, most infections are silent, but they can cause chronic pneumonia, especially in people with emphysema. Widespread disease can cause infection in the liver, spleen, bone marrow, and gastrointestinal tract.

diabetes who smoke are at even greater risk of having impaired circulation, which can lead to more foot infection issues.

DEFENSIVE MEASURES As with all health issues related to diabetes, good blood sugar control is the first line of defense against foot infections. Beyond that, giving your feet a little more attention can help keep them healthy. Follow these tips:

■ Wash your feet in warm water using a mild soap. However, don't soak your feet, because this can lead to dry skin.

■ Trim your toenails when needed. The best way is to clip straight across and then use an emery board to smooth any sharp edges. If you have difficulty doing this yourself, see a podiatrist regularly for a safe trim.

■ Rub lotion on your feet, but don't smear anything between your toes.

■ Closely inspect your feet every day for any signs of blisters, cuts, sores, and calluses. You may have to use a mirror to see the bottom of your feet. Anything suspicious should be taken care of immediately. Pay special attention to the spaces between your toes where hidden abrasions linger.

■ Don't walk around barefoot.

■ Wear socks or hosiery to help prevent blisters.

■ Get plenty of exercise to stimulate blood flow to your feet.

■ Find the right fit when shoe shopping. Look for your new shoes at the end of the day when your feet are at their biggest, and take time to get both feet measured by someone trained to fit shoes properly. Be sure your new shoes have plenty of wiggle room so you don't get blisters.

■ Don't smoke.

■ If you find a corn or callus, don't try to treat yourself, and don't use any commercial corn cures, because they can cause additional skin damage. See a podiatrist.

Chapter 19 Hospital-Acquired Infections

It may seem ironic, but the place where you go to be healed can make you sick. Hospitals are havens for infection-causing bugs, but by following a few practical tips, you can have a healthier hospital stay. After all, about the only thing you want to pick up from the hospital is a magazine from the gift shop.

Hospital-Acquired Infections (Nosocomial Infections)

CULPRIT Several different kinds of bacteria, and less often, viruses and fungi, are responsible for hospital-acquired infections. The most common infectors are the bacteria *Staphylococcus aureus*, *Pseudomonas aeruginosa*, and *Escherichia coli*.

INFECTION INFO When you go to the hospital, physicians, nurses, and other health-care workers have a variety of tools at their disposal to save your life or better your physical condition. Unfortunately, these same tools can harbor bacteria and other bugs that can cause infection. Catheters, surgical implements, breathing tubes, and even latex gloves can spread infection if not properly used.

The health-care workers themselves can spread infection if they're not vigilant about washing their hands and changing gloves every time they move from one patient to another. Hospital-acquired infections can also be the result of contaminated ventilation or water systems. However, the development of a hospital-acquired infection does not necessarily mean something was done incorrectly.

Urinary tract infections, surgical wound site infections, bloodstream infections, and pneumonia are the most common ill-

---

ARE YOU REALLY ALLERGIC TO PENICILLIN? PART II

Many people say they are allergic to penicillin in its various forms. When asked how their body reacts, they answer in a variety of ways, many of which don't indicate any allergy:

"I had a rash on my stomach made up of little red spots that didn't itch. It went away in a day."

A nonspecific rash such as this is not a good reason to avoid penicillins if they are needed. There is no difference in the risk of severe allergy with subsequent use whether this nonspecific rash occurred or not.

"I got a shot of penicillin to treat gonorrhea and I got real jittery and shaky a few minutes later. The shakiness lasted 15 minutes."

Some intramuscular forms of penicillin are combined with a local anesthetic to dull the pain of the injection. If the painkiller is absorbed, some self-limited symptoms such as this one may occur.

"I was told that I can't take cephalosporins, too."

Cephalosporin antibiotics are similar to penicillins and might, but don't usually, cross-react in situations of severe penicillin allergy. Most people will tolerate this class of antibiotics without issue, but the risks and benefits of the treatment should be considered before use.

nesses transmitted in hospitals. Nosocomial infections are so virulent for a couple of reasons. First, hospitals are full of sick people who bring with them a variety of infectious agents. Second, hospital patients do not have strong immune systems. Their bodies are hard at work trying to recover from an illness, injury, or surgery. And when the immune system is not in top condition, your body's defenses are down and it's easy for a new bug to invade.

WHO'S AT RISK The Centers for Disease Control and Prevention (CDC) estimates that almost two million Americans get hospital-acquired infections each year, and 90,000 of those people die from them. Anyone who spends time in the hospital is at risk for infection, but the chances are greater for those who stay in an intensive care unit.

DEFENSIVE MEASURES You can take many precautions to steer clear of infections while in the hospital. In fact, the CDC estimates at least one-third of hospital-acquired illnesses can be avoided. Being aware of your rights as a patient and following a few practical tips will go a long way toward ensuring you don't leave the hospital sicker than when you got there:

- **Wash up.** Do your duty by washing your hands or at least using a hand sanitizing gel that doesn't require water every time you use the restroom or handle anything that might be a germ carrier. Suspect items include soiled sheets, a bedpan, and used tissues.
- **Ask away.** Don't be afraid to ask your physicians, nurses, and nurse's aides if they have washed their hands.

- **Watch that wound.** Be sure to keep the dressing around a wound dry and clean. Let a nurse know immediately if it gets wet or begins to loosen.

- **Care for that catheter.** Treat your catheter site as a wound dressing and keep it clean and dry. If the dressing comes loose or if the drainage tube becomes dislodged, tell your nurse.

- **Be part of the team.** Be sure everyone involved in your care knows of any potential medical conditions, such as diabetes, that may affect your healing.

- **Know and follow the rules.** Follow your physician's instructions and ask questions if you're unsure about anything he or she has instructed you to do or not do.

- **Be sure well-wishers are well.** Tell family or friends who are sick to send you a get-well card instead of dropping by for a visit.

Index

I
Influenza virus, **1** 2–17, 33–36, 42, 47.
　　See also **B**ird flu; Flu.
Invasive H. flu, **4** 7–48

J
Jaundice, 42, 9 **2**, 94, 97, 159, 166

K
Koplik's spots, **4** 8–49

L
LaCrosse virus, 144
Lassa fever, 19
Legionella pneumophila, 81–83
Legionnaires' disease, 81–83
Leptospirosis, 1 78
Lesions, 41, 61, 67, 69, 124
Lice
　　body, 174–1 **75**
　　head, 125–1 27, 174
Listeria monocytogenes, 110–111,
　　143–147
Listeriosis, 110–111
Lockjaw. *See* Tetanus.
Lyme disease, 87–89, 177
Lymphadenitis, 1 02
Lymphangitis, 1 01–102
Lymphocytes, CD4 T, 6
Lymphocytic choriomeningitis (LCM), 178
Lyssavirus, 147

M
Mad cow disease, 21–23, 30
Malaria, 159–161
Measles, 48–50, 121
Meningitis, 28, 47, 52, 62, 111, 173, 178
　　bacterial, 143–147
　　viral, 124, 143, 150–152, 178
Monkeypox, 49
Mononucleosis, infectious, 75–77
Mumps, 50–52, 150
Muscle aches, 13, 26, 28, 34, 37, 73, 76,
　　82, 87, 111, 115, 119, 141, 159
Mycobacterium tuberculosis, 85

N
Nausea, 12, 33, 34, 42, 78, 82, 89, 92,
　　94, 97, 112, 115, 118, 119, 144,
　　157, 159, 162, 166, 179
Necrotizing fasciitis, 24–25

Neisseria
　　gonorrhoeae, 63, 90
　　meningitidis, 143–147
Night sweats, 86, 138
Noroviruses, 115, 116

O
Orchitis, 51
Osteomyelitis, 89–90

P
Papanicolaou (Pap) smear, 63
Paralysis, 53, 54, 87, 91, 103, 124, 143,
　　148
Parrot fever, 172–173
Parvovirus B19, 121–123
Pasteurella multocida, 167
Pediculus
　　humanus capitis, 125
　　humanus humanus, 174
Pelvic inflammatory disease (PID), 60, 64
Penicillium notatum, 46
Petechiae, 138
Pinworms, 127–130
Plague, 9, 16, 151
Plasmodium
　　falciparum, 159
　　malariae, 159
　　ovale, 159
　　vivax, 159
Pneumonia, 6, 13, 26, 27, 35, 36–39, 41,
　　43, 47, 49, 81, 172, 178, 183, 186
Polio, 52–55
Pontiac fever, 81, 82
Postherpetic neuralgia, 55
Prion proteins, 21, 23
Proteus mirabilis, 133
Pseudomembranous colitis, 9
Pseudomembranous enterocolitis, 9, 10
Pseudomonas aeruginosa, 185
Pyelonephritis, 134, 136–137

R
Rabies, 147–150, 167, 168, 169
Rash, 40, 42, 45, 48, 49, 55, 68, 76, 78,
　　87, 121, 122, 124, 131, 132, 141,
　　157, 164, 174, 175, 176, 178, 179,
　　186
Rat-bite fever, 178
Reiter's syndrome, 60–61, 107, 113
Respiratory distress, 26, 103, 140
Reye's syndrome, 35, 42, 43, 50